Be Iron Fit

Time-Efficient Training Secrets
for Ultimate Fitness | DON FINK

Second Edition

LYONS PRESS
Guilford, Connecticut
An imprint of Globe Pequot Press

Lyons Press is an imprint of Globe Pequot Press.

Ironman and Ironman Triathlon are registered trademarks of the World Triathlon Corporation. Active Release Technique and ART are registered trademarks.

Project editor: David Legere
Text design: Libby Kingsbury
Layout artist: Kirsten Livingston
Cover Photo: Jessi Stensland (www.gojessi.com) by Action Sports International
Illustrations: Tom Debiasse

The Library of Congress has cataloged the earlier edition as follows:

Library of Congress Cataloging-in-Publication Data
Fink, Don.
  Be iron-fit : time-efficient training secrets for ultimate fitness / Don Fink.
    p. cm.
  ISBN 1-59228-239-3 (trade paper)
  1. Ironman triathlons. 2. Triathlon—Training. I. Title.
  GV1060.73.F57 2004
  796.42' 57—dc22

                                                          2004000660

ISBN 978-1-59921-857-1

Printed in United States of America
10 9 8 7 6 5 4 3 2 1

To my inspiration, Melanie.

CONTENTS

Acknowledgments

I wish to thank the following individuals:

Steve Adler, Maria Aitken, Dave and Annette Aitkenhead, Mark Allen, Jodi Alper, Joseph Altomare, Martin Avidan, Justin Baum, Chris Baynes, M. Scott Boyles, Kellie Brown, Gordo Byrn, Ray and Eve Campeau, Spencer Conway, Carl Curran, Tim Daveler, Evan Del Colle, Peter Dominick, Jerome Dorsey, O. J. Espinosa, Barry Farber, Scott Gac, Ken Glah, Cathy Grote, Ryan Grote, GU Energy, Richard Haig, Jr., Chris Hernandez, Scott Horns, Nick Horton, John Howard, Kathleen Hughes, Peter Hyland, Troy Jacobson, Adrian Jones, Andrew Jones, Jeff Kellogg, Lynn Kellogg, Thomas Krauss, Jed Kwartler, Larry Laconi, Terry Laughlin, Lothar Leder, Paul Le Houillier, Paul Levine, Jeff Liccardi, Steve Listzwan, Laura Litwin, Donna Mallory, Dave Mantle, Dawn Marinelli, Eric Marquard, Tom McCarthy, Jamey McEwen, Matt Mizenko, Bernadette Murphy, Steve Noone, Chris Page, Bill Peters, Francis Quinn, Glenn Regenye, Sean Reilly, Katy Roberts, Milo Schaefer, Dr. John M. Schneider, Eric Siskind, Spencer Smith, Karen Smyers, The Sports People, Paul St. Pierre, Jessi Stensland, Steve Tarpinian, Scott Tinley, Steve Tomlinson, Peter Turek, Meg Waldron, Jan Wanklyn, Scott Weiler, and Charles Windus.

Introduction

The Ironman triathlon began over thirty years ago in Hawaii, when a dozen or so athletes combined a 2.4-mile ocean swim, a 112-mile bike race, and a 26.2-mile marathon into a single competition. This once-obscure race has not only flourished over the years, it has exploded into "Ironmania."

It is estimated that over 100,000 individuals will compete in an Iron-distance triathlon this year and that number continues to grow rapidly, drawing competitors from all walks of life. The World Triathlon Corporation (WTC), owners of the Hawaii Ironman, now sanction over 20 Ironman races around the world. And there are countless non-sanctioned races at the Iron-distance as well. Some of the WTC races sell out their 2,000 entry slots within hours after they go on sale—a full year before the actual race.

Ironmania is no less contagious in North America. USA Triathlon, the nation's governing body for the sport of triathlon, has more than doubled its membership to over 110,000 in only the last five years. Completing the Iron-distance, either in Hawaii or at one of the dozens of other Ironman-distance races, is the most widely held personal goal for these athletes. Doing so earns them the coveted title of "Ironman."

I completed my first Ironman in 1992, and was instantly bitten by the Iron-distance bug. The experience was so rewarding that it became my passion. Not only was I fascinated with the challenge of developing my knowledge and skills, but I also became enthusiastic about helping others achieve their Iron dream. I have now competed in over thirty Iron-distance races all over the world and have coached hundreds of athletes to become Ironmen.

I've written this book for the triathlete or endurance athlete who is either ready to take on the challenge of the Iron-distance, or to achieve superior fitness. If your goal is to complete your first Iron-distance triathlon, to set a new personal best time, or just to become IronFit, you have come to the right place.

You can benefit most from this book if you already have a base level of triathlon knowledge. Perhaps you have participated in some shorter distance triathlons, or in road racing, century rides, or swim competitions. Starting with this basic level of experience, I will take you step-by-step through everything you need to know to prepare for and successfully complete a full Iron-distance triathlon.

Even if you have already completed an Iron-distance triathlon, I will show you how to train smarter and more productively. You will approach your next race not only armed for a peak performance, but for a more rewarding one as well.

And for those who have no interest in actually competing in an Iron-distance triathlon but want to achieve the ultimate level of fitness, I will teach you what you need to know to become IronFit. You will learn to train like the most efficient Iron-distance triathletes and reach new heights of personal fitness.

With that said, the most common obstacle for aspiring Ironmen and Ironwomen is the time commitment. How can you manage your career and family life and still find time to become IronFit?

I have worked with athletes from a wide range of professions and lifestyles. I mentor a doctor who is on the job 10 hours a day, commutes another 2 hours, and has a spouse, three kids, and Little League games and recitals to attend. I also mentor a house builder who has many of the same demands on his time, plus he carries Sheetrock up a ladder all day, zapping him of the energy he needs to train. The doctor and the house builder have more in common than their busy schedules. Both are now Ironmen.

Years ago I worked over 60 hours a week running a major investment business with a large staff and billions of dollars under management. In addition to overseeing my company's offices in New Jersey and Washington, D.C., I was required to attend meetings at the New York headquarters, travel all over the country to see clients and attend conferences, and host client dinners in the evenings and on weekends. I often struggled to find training time. And when I did find it, it was often at odd hours and in unfamiliar surroundings.

The demands of my wife's career were much the same. So just figuring out how to care for our three rescued greyhounds, keep up our home, and attend the usual family functions was a challenge.

I realized that in order to compete in triathlon I would need to learn how to train efficiently and manage my time effectively. I started by learning many of the most successful training techniques from the top coaches and athletes, such as Mark Allen, Barry Farber, John Howard, Troy Jacobson, Terry Laughlin, Dave Scott, Karen Smyers, Steve Tarpinian, and many others. Over time, I built upon the techniques of these experts through my own experimentation and experiences. Most importantly, I brought my knowledge of efficiency and time management from the business world and applied it to my training. It was an unbeatable combination.

I discovered the counterintuitive nature of training, that "No pain, no gain" is a myth. More is not always better. In fact, sometimes more is just more, and worse, sometimes more is actually less. I learned to work with my body, not against it. And I was able to achieve levels of performance I never thought possible.

I only have time to coach about fifty athletes personally. Through this book, I hope to reach out to as many athletes as possible. I want to help you to accomplish your Iron dream.

I will show you how to achieve your goal, just as I have for hundreds of other successful Iron-distance triathletes. In *Be IronFit* I combine my time-efficient training methods, my time-management techniques, and my unique knowledge and experience of Iron-distance triathlons to give you everything you need to know to be successful and achieve your Iron dream.

What's more, it's going to be enjoyable. That's right. You will be amazed at how much fun you will have on your journey. After all, swimming, biking, and running should be fun, shouldn't they? When you train smart and have a positive approach, they are.

I will not give you a lot of complicated science and technical lingo: just straight talk and a clear path to the Iron dream. I will explain all of the key elements and provide methods to build on these elements and sustain your training over your IronFit journey: how to train, how to manage your time, how to prioritize, how to select the best races, race strategy, equipment choices, technique, mental training, motivation, and much more.

I will present three specific 30-week training plans to prepare you to be IronFit. In each program I will tell you the exact workouts you need to complete each day to accomplish your goal: the exact step-by-step secrets to make your dream a reality. After reading this book and learning its time-management secrets you will be in a position to determine realistically how much time you can spend on training, and then select the 30-week program best suited for you.

If you are a busy person with the desire to be IronFit, this book is for you. I will explain the most efficient way to train, the best time-management techniques, and provide all of the information you will need to know to see you through to your Iron dream.

Take the next step—turn the page—and I will see you at the finish line.

CHAPTER 1

The IronFit Dream

"The soul should always stand ajar, ready to
welcome the ecstatic experience."

—Emily Dickinson

I am continually amazed at the number of people harboring the dream of completing an Iron-distance triathlon. And that amazement extends to the even larger number of people who admire Iron-distance finishers and seek to attain "Iron" fitness, even though they might not want to compete in a full-length event. People from all walks of life are drawn to this incredible athletic challenge. The Iron-distance continues to touch so many people in a deep and emotional way.

Now, after many years of racing Iron-distance triathlons and coaching others to do the same, I have come to realize that there are really only two kinds of triathletes: those who admit that their ultimate goal is to complete an Iron-distance triathlon and those who don't say it but secretly desire it just the same. The Iron-distance is the heart and soul of multisport racing. It is what drives every triathlete at some point.

Nowhere is this more true than in the United States. USA Triathlon, the national governing body for the sport, currently claims 110,000 members and is experiencing robust growth in its membership, year after year. This is directly related to the surging popularity of Iron-distance racing. All of the U.S.-based Iron-distance races are seeing substantial growth in the number of competitors every year.

Some of the most popular races, like Ironman USA in Lake Placid, New York and Ironman Florida in Panama City, Florida, sell out their 2,500 entry slots in hours if not minutes. This is particularly significant, as they offer their slots a full year before the actual competition. If you plan to participate in these extremely popular races, you must make your plans a full year in advance. Fortunately, there are several other great races, where the competition for entry is not as intense.

Why the allure? What makes the goal of completing an Iron-distance triathlon so powerful for so many athletes? It all begins with how we first learn about the Ironman.

The first phase is Nonbelief. For most of us, the first triathlon we see is the Hawaii Ironman on television, either those famous segments years ago on ABC's Wide World of Sports, or NBC's fully dedicated programs in more recent years. And the first thought that comes to your mind as you stare at the screen is, "That's impossible."

You learn the exact distances: a 2.4-mile ocean swim, followed by a 112-mile bike race, and then a full 26.2-mile marathon—back-to-back and all in the same day. Then you hear about the weather conditions in Hawaii—the severe heat and powerful winds—and you think, "People can't really do that." Perhaps you had always thought a marathon was the ultimate test of athletic endurance. Surely something so much longer and more challenging is impossible for the human body.

The second phase is Realization. You watch more of the race. You see the individual athletes and their heroic struggles to the finish. You can see their incredible sense of pride and accomplishment. You get pulled into it. "Wow, there are people who can actually do this!" The impossible starts to become the possible . . . at least it becomes possible for these people.

The third phase is Curiosity. You start asking questions. Why do these people do this? What motivates them? How do they do it? How do they train?

Then comes the final stage, The Dream. You ask yourself the big question: I wonder if I could ever do it? I wonder if I could ever be an Ironman?

That's it! This is the fascination of the Iron-distance triathlon, and the reason why so many harbor the Iron-distance dream. In a short period, you go from believing that something is definitely not possible to believing that it is possible. In fact, you begin to think that it might even be possible for you.

This is the allure of the Iron-distance, and it transcends athletics. We realize that we may be too quick to judge what is possible and what is not. Perhaps other "impossibilities" in our lives are also much more possible than we had previously thought. Perhaps if we can do this race, something we once thought impossible, we will prove to ourselves that our potential is far greater than we had ever imagined.

Now the good news/bad news. First the bad news: While many are touched by The Dream of completing an Iron-distance triathlon, far fewer act on it. It's so easy to find a reason not to attempt it. It seems too risky. The training is probably too complicated. You don't have enough time. There is too much to learn. And so on. My purpose in this book, of course, is to answer every one of these concerns and provide you with everything you need to know to live The Dream.

Now for the good news: For those who do act on The Dream, the rewards are greater than they had ever anticipated. Competitors who complete the Iron-distance look back on the moment when they crossed the finish line as one of the most significant and powerful moments in their lives. Not only that, most of them also look back on the entire journey of becoming an Ironman as one of the most rewarding periods of their lives. That's right. The training is not a painful, grinding process. If you know what to do and you have the right program for you, every day of your journey toward becoming an Ironman is exciting and rewarding. It is a great thrill to have that Iron-distance race day on the calendar and to get up every day anxious to implement the plan that will make The Dream a reality.

I was never the same person again after my first Iron-distance triathlon, and neither is anyone else. It does something wonderful to you, and it's not just the thrill of crossing the finish line. It starts when you make the commitment to the race and it continues well beyond. It's an amazing journey of self-discovery that carries on after you cross the finish line and continues for the rest of your life.

After you complete an Iron-distance triathlon, it will always be on your shortlist of lifetime accomplishments. You can't help it—it will be. If someone asks you, "What's the most amazing thing you've ever done?" you will immediately see yourself finishing the Ironman.

So for all those out there with The Dream in the back of your head, I am talking to you. You can do it. You will never regret doing it. You will almost definitely regret, deeply regret, not doing it. You need only to decide to take the journey, the most amazing journey of your life. This is your road map.

Why It Is So Difficult to Achieve the IronFit Dream

Having The Dream is the first step. But then what? People who are driven enough to have The Dream often have demanding careers, families, and other responsibilities. Just maintaining family and career is more than enough to fill up your days. How can you possibly add this major undertaking? There just don't seem to be enough hours in the day.

And even if you did have the time, how would you train for something like this? What if you only have experience at one of the three sports and are a novice at the others?

The good news is it's doable. If you know how, it's very doable. Just look at the vast majority of Iron-distance finishers. They are not full-time athletes; they're people just like you. They have families, careers, and all of life's usual responsibilities. The secret to accomplishing The Dream is combining highly efficient training with effective time management.

The three key components to the Iron-distance equation are: (1) highly efficient training, (2) highly effective time-management skills, and (3) "been there, done that" knowledge.

This is what I have been doing for years, mentoring athletes to their Iron-distance goal by helping them to master these essential components. Most of my athletes have demanding careers, most have families and other important responsibilities, but all were successful in their goal of completing an Iron-distance triathlon. And what's more, they all greatly enjoyed the experience. Sure, there are up days and down days along the way. But for the most part, everyone enjoyed each step in his or her journey.

I am not a believer in the "no pain, no gain" philosophy. I believe in training smart and training safe. The approaches and methods I describe below will allow you to maintain balance in your life, as well as derive great pleasure and a sense of accomplishment each step along the way.

What We Can Learn from the Great Ones

Not all professional triathletes are the same. Sure, there are many who are unmarried and fully sponsored; all they need to focus on is training and racing. But this is not universal. Some pro triathletes have lives much more "normal" than you would expect. Some have spouses and children. Many have to balance their training with demands on their time from sponsors, coaching, public appearances, and travel. Two of the greatest and most successful Ironman champions ever could be described this way.

Karen Smyers is probably the most successful and versatile athlete in the history of triathlon. She has consistently won races at every distance from sprint to Ironman. In addition to being the 1995 Ironman World Champion, she has won three World Championships and six USA Pro Championships at the Olympic distance (1.5K swim, 40K bike, and 10K run). Quite simply, she has been one of the most dominant women in triathlon over the last twenty years.

And yet Karen's life was not so simple as just training and racing. At the time of this writing, Karen and her husband Michael had a young daughter, and they were committed and loving parents. Karen served as the pro athlete representative to USA Triathlon. In addition, she coached, made public appearances, and fulfilled various obligations to her sponsors.

And there's more: Karen Smyers has had more than her share of obstacles to overcome along the way. In addition to several serious accidents and injuries from bike crashes, Karen has survived thyroid cancer. As with everything else, Karen handled these challenges with grace and good humor.

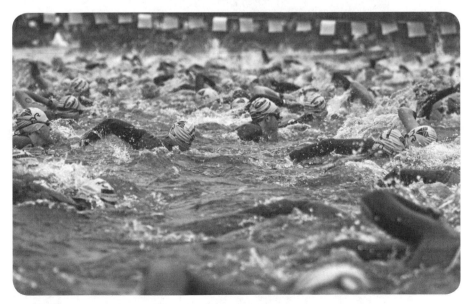

Photo Credit: Lynn Kellogg/www.trilifephotos.com.

When I asked her what one word came to her mind to explain her incredible success, she quickly answered, "Perseverance." Karen would say that she was not a born triathlete. As she explains it, "I was never a standout right from the very beginning in any of the sports—swimming, cycling, or running. So for sure, I think a lot of it is just sticking with it, and I think it's important to like what you are doing, so that you don't have a false motivation. If you like what you're doing, you are more apt to stick to it."

Lothar Leder is not only one of the world's most winning Ironman triathletes, he can also claim the unique distinction of being the first athlete in the history of Ironman to break 8 hours. Like Roger Bannister, the first

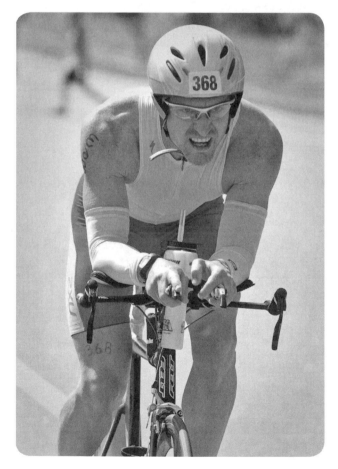

Scott Boyles, married, father of two, attorney . . . Iron-distance triathlete. Photo Credit: © 2009 *Birds Eye View.*

runner ever to run a mile under 4 minutes, Lothar has secured immortality in his sport thanks to this single accomplishment. There can only be one first, and Lothar will always be that person.

But it doesn't stop there. Lothar has been one of the most successful and exciting triathletes of our time. In addition to being a multiple Challenge Roth (formerly known as Ironman Europe) winner, he has won dozens of major races around the world. Like Karen Smyers, he has proven his ability to win anytime, anywhere, and at any distance. Also like Karen, Lothar has a friendly, outgoing personality that makes him a great example for our sport.

But Lothar Leder's life is not only focused on training and racing. At the time of this writing, Lothar and his wife Nicole, also a champion triathlete, had a young daughter to care for. They too had sponsorship, appearance, and coaching responsibilities, as well as the pressures of extensive traveling.

When I asked Lothar the same question—What one word comes to mind to explain your success?—he replied, "Will." He said, "I have the will to train, the will to sacrifice, and the will to win." He quickly followed up on this, however, adding, "I am also very organized." He explained he learned good time-management skills as a young swimmer, and this has helped him a great deal as a triathlete.

Why do I share these insights from the great Karen Smyers and Lothar Leder? Because of what they identify as the keys to their success: perseverance, will, and organization. These same elements will be the key to our success at triathlon. This book will teach you how to train properly, how to manage your time, and how to achieve your IronFit goal. It will also help you to tap into your will and perseverance, traits that will assure your success.

CHAPTER 2

Effective Time Management

"What you do during your working
hours determines what we have;
what you do during our leisure hours
determines who we are."

—*George Eastman*

There are two sides to our Iron-distance training equation. In addition to learning to train as effectively and efficiently as possible, we also need to find time for our workouts in our busy schedules. In this chapter, I will present many of the time-management techniques that have helped hundreds of Ironmen to succeed. I will then present the first of several IronFit athlete profiles that will appear throughout. Each will present the personal time-management tips of successful Iron-distance triathletes, from all walks of life, but with one big similarity: They are all extremely busy people who once started with an Iron-distance dream.

Having worked with hundreds of triathletes, I have found the following five time-management techniques to be the most successful and widely utilized. These are the "Big Five":

1. Train Time, Not Miles

2. Indoor Training

3. Lunchtime Workouts

4. Masters Swimming Sessions

5. Early Bird Workouts

1. Train Time, Not Miles

Some of our time-management tips are quick fixes, while others are going to take some work. This first one is definitely a quick fix.

A great way to manage your training time is simply to train in terms of time, not in distance. While we can estimate how long a particular distance is going to take to run or cycle, many other factors come into play, and these estimates can easily be off. So instead of going for a 5-mile run, go for a 45-minute run. Schedule it right into your daily calendar, just as you would any other appointment. All of the guesswork is eliminated.

For various reasons, the vast majority of athletes tend to plan their training in terms of distance. If we can break this habit and make this minor change, we can do a much better job of managing our training time. As we will see in Chapter 7, all of the training plans in this book are expressed in time, not distance.

In addition to improved time management, there are many other benefits of time-based training. For one, there is no longer any need to measure out training courses. You can just head out the door, run in whatever direction you feel like, and then turn around at the halfway point and run back.

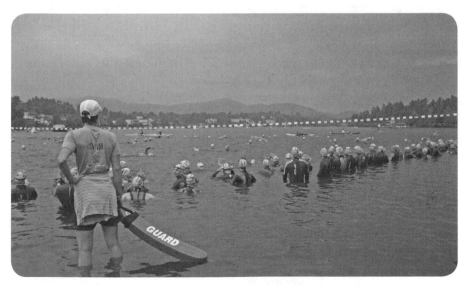

Photo Credit: Lynn Kellogg/www.trilifephotos.com.

This is particularly advantageous for the business traveler. No matter where you are, you can run out of your hotel and make your route up as you go. This has been a great adventure for me over the years: It was always a fun way to explore a new city or country. Be safe though; once in New Zealand I made an unfortunate turn and came face-to-face with an angry bull.

As we will see in Chapter 6, there is another major advantage to time-oriented runs and rides: They fit in perfectly with heart rate–based training. In heart rate training, we are looking to maximize our time spent training at a particular heart rate. For these workouts it is necessary to track time, not distance.

2. Indoor Training

Indoor workouts, for instance on treadmills or stationary bikes, can often be more time-efficient than outdoor training. Properly integrated into an Iron-distance training program, these workouts can actually provide more effective training overall. This is especially important because it helps us accomplish both of our goals in this book: to manage our time better, and to derive greater benefit from the time we dedicate to training.

I am not suggesting that you do all of your training indoors. There are definite advantages to outdoor training. Certain aspects of training, such as getting the "true feel," can best be accomplished outdoors. Bike skills such as climbing, descending, and cornering are examples of this. But mixing in some indoor training can help you manage your time better and make your training more efficient.

If you can afford to install training equipment in your home, or if you are lucky enough to have it available near your place of work, it can greatly decrease your "workout commuting" time. Long drives to the fitness center add time to our training and increase the likelihood that we will miss workouts.

Indoor training allows us to control our conditions. No more delays due to bad weather. Those living in northern regions with harsh winters can especially benefit. Snow, rain, ice, severe cold, and limited daylight hours can be a real challenge to training. Training indoors may even help to keep head colds away and keep you healthier as well.

Another plus is that indoor training can increase the time you spend with your family. Instead of heading out the door and away from your loved ones, you can set up your stationary bike in the family room and be with them. Becoming an Ironman and spending time with your family do not have to be conflicting goals. Many of the Ironmen I have worked with have become masters at doing two things at once. This is one of their most popular techniques.

In addition I have heard from many athletes that training seems to have a positive effect on others. Surely your children must gain something positive from seeing you training and working so hard toward a goal.

3. Lunchtime Workouts

Midday training sessions are overlooked by most athletes, but they offer an enormous time-management opportunity. Most people have at least 45 minutes to an hour available for lunch. Some companies offer fitness facilities on the premises or at least nearby, and even if they don't, there may be off-site fitness centers or pools available. This is a great asset that you should take advantage of. If you can get in two or three lunchtime training sessions per week, you have completed a substantial portion of your weekly training. Of the three 30-Week IronFit Training Programs I present in Chapter 7, even the one with the largest time commitment averages only 12 hours of training per week. Just think, if you can get in four midday training sessions per week, you will knock off 25% to 33% of your total training time.

Another advantage of lunchtime training is that it still is fairly early in the day, so your energy level tends to be high. Just remember to have a healthy midmorning snack to ensure that you will be ready to go.

Midday training is also a great stress reducer. I have always found that these sessions revitalize me and prepare me for a calm and productive afternoon. Currently I leave my office at noon several days a week for a nearby pool. I can get in a crisp swim session and be back at my desk (with a healthy snack) by 1:15 p.m., refreshed and ready to put in a productive afternoon.

4. Masters Swimming Sessions

A Masters swim program is one of the most valuable training assets you can tap to accomplish your IronFit Dream. If there is a program available in your area you should definitely look into it. This is especially true if you do not have a swimming background.

United States Masters Swimming (USMS) is a national nonprofit organization that offers organized workouts, competitions, and other programs; despite its name, the organization is open to swimmers aged 18 and over. Masters swimming programs meet at a specific time, so you can schedule them into your calendar just like any other appointment. Most programs are scheduled for either early morning or evening, so they fit around most athletes' work schedules.

It can be tough to get yourself to the pool and then push through a workout on your own—especially after a long day at work. One of the great things about Masters is that all you have to do is motivate yourself to show up. The rest of the workout takes care of itself. You have people to swim with and motivate you, and you have a coach on deck who can offer feedback on your technique. Masters swimming is also great fun. You will meet motivated people just like yourself, some of whom will share your IronFit dream. You will meet new friends and training buddies.

In the Masters program that I coach, I find many athletes join the program with the desire to improve their swimming so that they can successfully complete an Iron-distance triathlon. The newcomers are often amazed to find dozens of other Ironmen in the class, plus many other aspiring Ironmen. They go there for swimming but what they find is an amazing support system for triathlon.

If you are not aware of a Masters swimming program in your area, check out the Web site of United States Masters (www.usms.org) for programs in your area.

Don't despair if you find that there isn't a Masters swimming program in your area that fits your schedule and needs. A Masters swim program is a nice-to-have, but by no means a need-to-have. Chapter 11 will provide you with information for improving your swim technique, special drills to help you become more efficient, and guidance on exactly what you need to do when you go to the pool.

5. Early Bird Workouts

OK, now the big one! I mentioned that some of our time-management tips would be quick fixes and some might be a bit more challenging. For many of us, this one is the most challenging to accomplish.

One of the most common time-management recommendations you will hear from Ironmen is to get your training in early in the day. Depending on your work situation, wake up early on weekdays and get at least some of your daily training completed. If you plan to do it all after work you risk not doing it at all. Meetings run late, people drop in, computers go down; you name it, it happens. The best way to make sure that you get it done is to do it early. Even 1 hour before work each weekday means 5 solid hours of training time.

The same applies to weekend training. Wake up early and get it done. Don't allow yourself to ease into the day because, again, you risk not getting it in. Too many things can happen—family responsibilities, friends stopping by, a call from your boss to work over the weekend.

The best strategy is to get training done early and thus clear the deck for whatever comes up. This is especially important with your family. It will make a big difference if you can say, "I'll be out training in the morning, but after 10 a.m. I'm all yours." They are going to be much more supportive.

Another reason to get into the habit of training in the morning is to take advantage of your highest energy level of the day. Between your family and work responsibilities and your IronFit training, you are going to be tired toward the end of the day. Your energy level is usually best in the early morning.

I know what some of you are going to say: "But I'm not a morning person." I understand this reaction, because I felt the same way. I was the ultimate non-morning person for most of my life. What I found over time, however, was that "stuff happens" during the day, and far too often I would miss my workout. I decided to give morning workouts a trial for one month. It was tough. I found it hard to get going in the morning and I felt tired much earlier in the day. Gradually, however, I got used to it. And once I did, guess what? My training sessions actually became more productive. Once my system became accustomed to my new schedule, I found that I actually had a much higher energy level in the morning than in the evening.

It was easier mentally as well. My training was completed before work and family emergencies had a chance to pop up. I didn't go through the day with the challenging workout hanging over my head. And no matter how the day went, I always had that great feeling of accomplishment right from the start.

I used to train for Iron-distance events while I was also working 60 hours a week. I did my cycling or running session (or both) in the morning before work. (By the way, I used to arrive at work wide awake and ready to go, while my coworkers were still drinking coffee and wiping away the sleepers!) Then I swam on one or two evenings per week, on my way home from work.

Weekends were similar. I left early Saturday morning for my long bike ride and was back home in the late morning with the rest of the day open for family, relaxation, errands, etc. On Sunday, I got my long run in first thing and then, in the late afternoon, I got in my third swim of the week.

Let's be honest with ourselves. None of us was born an "evening person." We just became accustomed to that lifestyle. If your desire is great enough—and if you are reading this book, it is—you can become accustomed to a new lifestyle. Ask yourself: Do I want to be the person who is always up to date on Leno or Letterman, or do I want to live my dream of being IronFit?

For all you "I'm not a morning person" types, the following Take Action Challenge is for you:

TAKE ACTION CHALLENGE: 21 DAYS OF MORNING WORKOUTS

Commit to morning training for the next 21 days. Write out a schedule, or mark your planner or calendar, with the time you will wake each day and do your workout. Each day, upon completing the workout, check it off in your calendar. When it feels difficult to get up some mornings, remind yourself that this will only be for 21 days, and then think about how you will feel someday when you cross the finish line at an Iron-distance triathlon.

This Take Action Challenge presents a proven tool to help athletes make this important lifestyle change. A lot of people try training in the morning and decide after a few days that it doesn't feel right, so they go back to their old ways. The 3-week approach works because it is short enough to commit to as an experiment, but long enough to allow the athlete to adjust to the new lifestyle. You get through the transition by telling yourself that it's only for 21 days, but ultimately, you make the adjustment during this period and are able to continue comfortably with morning training after the 3-week trial.

What if you try it for 21 days and still can't make morning training work for you? Don't despair. While mornings work best for most people there are notable exceptions, busy athletes who have been able to accomplish The Dream with little or no morning training. One such triathlete is Evan Del Colle, who is the subject of our first IronFit Profile. Evan feels that despite his long days filled with career and family responsibilities, his energy levels are best in the evening.

Following is our first of many IronFit Profiles. Each profile will include a description of the individual's lifestyle and personal situation, as well as his or her personal time-management tips and secrets. These profiles will present many additional time management techniques, beyond the "Big Five" presented earlier in this chapter. Hopefully you will find the answers to your specific time-management challenges in the stories of these amazing people.

IRONFIT PROFILE

Evan Del Colle (written in 2004)

If Evan Del Colle can do it, anyone can. Evan is living proof that the premise of this book is true. With effective time management and efficient training, an individual can achieve balance in their life and still find success at the Iron-distance. As a child, Evan suffered a brain tumor, which left him with partial paralysis. As you can imagine, he had more than his share of uphill battles over the years. Today, at forty-two years old, Evan has a great marriage, two wonderful kids, and a successful career with one of the nation's most prestigious companies, and yes . . . Evan is an "Ironman."

Evan Del Colle completed his first Iron-distance triathlon (The Great Floridian in Clermont, Florida) in 1998 and more recently his second, the 2001 Ironman USA in Lake Placid, New York. He has a demanding career with Chase-J.P. Morgan Bank, one of the largest financial institutions in the world. He commutes into New York City each weekday from his home in New Jersey. Evan leaves home at 6 a.m. each weekday morning and returns at 6:30 p.m., for a total of about 63 hours per week.

Evan sleeps about 4 hours per night during the week and about 6 on weekends, for a weekly total of about 32 hours.

As important as his work responsibilities are to him, Evan's family is of course his first priority. He has two children, eleven and seven, and is actively involved in their lives. He coaches his son's basketball team, which takes about 8 hours per week. Evan also shares some of the responsibilities for caring for an elderly family member.

Evan trains 10 to 15 hours per week on average during the year, with peak Iron-distance training of about 20 hours per week. He trains mostly in the evening, although he plans ahead so that if he has a conflict in the evening he will get his training in during the morning or at lunchtime. He belongs to a health and fitness club near work and tries to use it as much as possible to take time pressure off his evening workouts.

For Evan the key is planning. He makes three copies of his weekly training plan and keeps it in three key places so that he is always sure to plan around his schedule. Surprisingly, Evan tries to schedule his training activities around family activities and work, not the other way around. As determined as he is to get his daily training session in, he gives higher priority to his family and work responsibilities. This would seem to imply that training frequently gets squeezed out of the picture in favor of other priorities, but this is rarely the case. Because of his consistent planning and his flexibility about when he trains, Evan usually gets it all in every day.

Evan's wife Kathy has been very supportive of Evan's athletic pursuits. Like many spouses of first-time Iron-distance triathletes, she assumed that Evan's first Ironman would probably be his last. He would do this "Ironman thing" and then get it out of his system and move on to a more normal life. As often happens, however, his first Iron-distance triathlon was only the first. The experience of taking the Iron-distance journey and successfully making it to the finish line changes a person. The individual crossing the line is not the same one that started the journey. More often than not, this initial Iron-distance journey leads to additional journeys.

Well Evan's wife came to understand this, and she along with their two children are totally supportive of their husband/father and proud of the fact that the man in their lives is a member of one of the most elite groups on earth—an "Ironman."

How does he do it? Brain tumor survivor. Paralysis survivor. Loving father and husband. Successful in his career. "Ironman." Evan says it's his attitude. "I'm always in the game," he says. "I am in the game to win or lose, but I'm always in the game." This is the attitude of Evan Del Colle. He doesn't talk about hardships or set-backs. He looks at life as a challenge. He packs every element of life into every day and he truly enjoys the journey along the way.

Following are some more of Evan's favorite time-saving tips:

Cat Naps: Commuting by train provides Evan with a great opportunity to catch up on sleep when he needs to. If you try this, don't forget to set the alarm on your watch to make sure you don't miss your stop!

Enjoy the Challenge: Evan doesn't look at his time constraints as a problem; he views them as a challenge. "How do I fit a 2-hour training session into my day?" Evan asks. "It's tough sometimes, but I almost always do it." Evan prides himself on winning this daily challenge.

Train in Time Not Miles: Evan agrees with the training concept of measuring your workouts in time not miles. Instead of going for an 8-mile run, Evan goes for a 60-minute run. There is no need to measure courses, and no miscalculations occur. Training by time, not miles, is a natural for effective time management.

Indoor Training: Evan often uses indoor training methods, such as a treadmill or stationary bike, and finds it to be more time effective, in part because there are no weather delays and less time needed to get dressed and prepare equipment, especially in cold weather.

AN IRONFIT MOMENT

"Window of Opportunity"

The following was written by Evan Del Colle before his first Iron-distance in 1998. Evan successfully completed The Greater Floridian Triathlon a few days later and became an Ironman.

This is the imaginary window, too hard to open and too hard to close. This my friend is the window of time. 168 hours per week, sounds reasonable and yes indeed, exact!

However, 24 hours a day and utilizing those hours creates that illusionary "window of time." Take myself, commuting to and from lower Manhattan. That's 18 hours a week—the window is already closing. And I forgot to add that, working in a large financial institution, I donate 40 to 50 hours. So getting out my calculator, that leaves me with 100 hours.

Now, let's not forget the essentials, or SESA: sleeping, eating, showering, and all other complements performed in looking and feeling good. So you're slowly closing the window and we haven't yet spoken about training hours, but we know that SESA is going to rob you of at least 35 hours a week. I kind of figure a triathlete will invent some device that allows you to eat while you sleep, or sleep while you eat, but this is only 1998.

Now, for the intelligent and efficient one, who would say, "Sleep on the job." Sounds great, but bad execution, so let's ignore that one.

By having at least a third-grade math proficiency, you can see how the 168 hours a week is now down to 65. You can see where I am headed, and in general terms to the best of my ability, one will say, "That's life, deal with it." (Probably said by somebody with a beer in one hand and a remote in the other.)

Now, where were we, ah yes, I have a family that I didn't even debit from my balance! So family life, coaching commitments, and just hanging out with friends leave me with a dwindling 30 hours. That window slowly closing each week is my time to train. Now that's nearly 20% of the week, but that 20% is always robbed by an emergency, or a commitment, something unexpected, each and every week. So back to the "true" time. That 30 hours is actually in the neighborhood of 20. Make those 1,200 minutes count, damn it!

So with the 20 hours I have in the reserve, week after week, I pound my body, test my body, and be the best I can be in my training quest. As we watch the window close, we can say, well time is money, but that gets into another story. So please don't ask, I have to train!

CHAPTER 3

The Essential Workouts

*"To give anything less than your best
is to sacrifice the gift."*

—Steve Prefontaine

In this chapter I will present the essential workouts that make up a successful IronFit training program. This is not the training program itself, but the basic units with which we will build each week of our program. In Chapter 4 we will discuss how to arrange these individual sessions within a week, but first I will describe these key workouts, discuss how to approach each of them, and explain why each of these sessions is important to our overall program.

The Long Ride and the Long Run

The two most important workouts of the week are the Long Bike and the Long Run.

Not only are these the most important, they are also the most time consuming, so given our topic, they are a great place to start.

First the good news: To complete an Iron-distance triathlon, you do not have to train by running and riding for several hours every day. I recommend only that you "go long" once each week, and that these rides and runs only exceed 4 hours and 2 hours, respectively, during the final peak weeks leading up to your race date. If you can find the time to get these sessions in, you can do an Iron-distance triathlon.

Now the not-so-good (but expected) news: If you want to race long, you have to train long. You need to teach your body how to do it by doing it. The trick is to allow your body to adapt to it very gradually. Gradually build up the duration of your Long Rides and Long Runs.

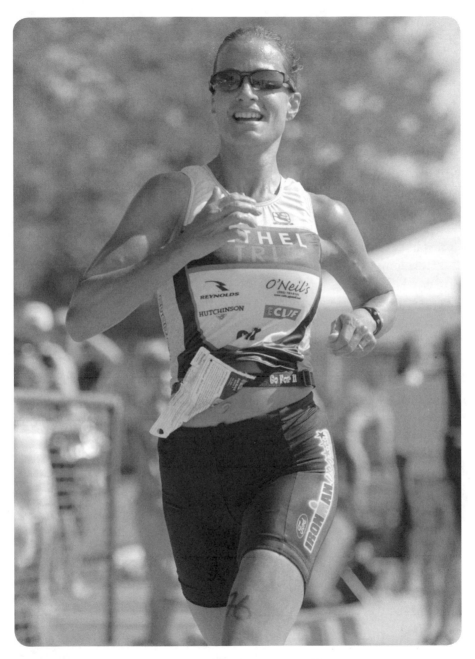

Kellie Brown, married, veterinarian . . . Iron-distance triathlete.
Photo Credit: Capstone Photography.

It is important to understand that these long rides and runs don't need to be performed at a high level of effort. I recommend that you complete them at a very comfortable, aerobic pace (65–85% of maximum heart rate). There is no need to push hard in these workouts. The pace I recommend is adequate to train your aerobic system, and that is what we're after. If you push harder in these workouts you risk burnout and injury. We will explore this further in Chapter 6.

For most people who work 9 to 5 (or more likely 8 to 6), the best time for these workouts is Saturday morning for the Long Bike and Sunday for the Long Run. For most, the best way is to do it early. If you put it off, something will always come up. Get up early and get it out of the way so you can deal with your family responsibilities and all the other things that need to be done on the weekend.

How long does the Long Bike need to be? During the 10-week Build Phase, which falls in the middle of the training programs presented in Chapter 7, you should gradually build up this ride to 4 hours. Not too bad! Get everything set the night before. Set the alarm for a little before 6 or 7 a.m., and you will be back by 10 or 11 a.m., hardly even missed.

In the final 10 weeks before the race, when you start your final Peak Phase, you will gradually add time to your ride each week, bringing it up to 5 or 6 hours at the 3-weeks-to-go point. Even this isn't too bad. If you can get out the door by 6 a.m., you will be back by noon with a good portion of the day ahead of you.

How long does the Long Run need to be? During the Build Phase, this run should be gradually built up to 2 hours. In the final 10 weeks, when you start your final Peak Phase, you then gradually add time to your run each week, bringing it up to 3 hours at the 3-weeks-to-go point.

As with the Long Ride, get up and get these Long Runs in early to make sure they get done.

Transition Workouts

Transition Workouts (aka "Brick" Workouts) are sessions that include one or more quick transitions between two sports. Usually they involve a bike ride followed by a quick transition to running gear and a run.

After you have built your Long Bike and Long Run sessions into your training schedule, this is the next most beneficial training element to include. Triathlon is not three separate sports; it's really just one sport. Each sport affects the others. Your swim impacts your bike, your bike impacts your run, etc. You are not training to run a marathon; you are training to run a marathon after you have cycled 112 miles. There is a difference.

You need to teach your body to run well despite the effects of a long bike ride. As a result, "running fresh" only has limited training benefits. You need to teach your body to run when it's not fresh. That's what Transition Workouts will bring to your training.

High Intensity Runs and Rides

In addition to "going long" each week in both cycling and running, it is also helpful to go fast. In these workouts you want to go faster than your expected Iron-distance race pace and push your heart rate into the anaerobic zone (see Chapter 6).

Most athletes actually do too much High Intensity training. Because it is important for short-distance triathlons, many athletes incorporate a relatively large percentage of High Intensity work in their Iron-distance training programs. As we shall see, in a perfect Iron-distance race your heart rate would never reach anaerobic levels; so it's questionable why you need any High Intensity training at all. In fact, you don't. It is quite possible to complete an Iron-distance triathlon on nothing but aerobic training. The reverse statement is difficult to make. Aerobic training is the key to Iron-distance racing.

Ideally, I recommend that you limit High Intensity training to only about 5% to 10% of your total Iron-distance training. Opinions vary on this point, but this is what I have found to work best for most.

Well, then why should we include High Intensity training at all? The following are some of the benefits of including a small portion of High Intensity training in your Iron-distance training program. High Intensity training:

- Prepares your body to recover more efficiently from intense efforts and settle back into your aerobic zone. There are many times during an Iron-distance race when your heart rate may become anaerobic, e.g., at the swim start, when climbing a hill, or when transitioning from one sport to another. This type of training helps you recover from these efforts.

- Builds overall strength.

- Increases leg turnover.

- Adds variety to training.

High RPM Spin Sessions

The High RPM (revolutions per minute) Spin workout is an important training session to develop cycling technique.

Many beginners first approach cycling by pushing down on one pedal while pulling up on the other. As will be discussed in Chapter 11, this approach is inefficient and can actually be dangerous and cause leg injuries. What we want to do is "spin" our pedals in a circle, applying roughly equal force on the pedal throughout each revolution.

We will use the High RPM Spin session primarily to help develop this technique. Additionally, since this tends to be a less strenuous type of workout, we will also use it in certain situations for active recovery. Active recovery refers to lower intensity workouts, which allow the athlete to continue training while recovering from prior more taxing efforts.

In the High RPM Spin session we will use a relatively easy gear and spin the pedals at 100 or more RPM. More advanced cyclists may feel comfortable spinning at 110 or more, but if you are still developing your spin technique it's best to keep it right at, or just above, 100 RPM.

While doing this workout, you want to consciously think about applying equal force to the pedals throughout each full revolution. If you focus on this in training, your good technique will become automatic in your racing.

One great way to develop efficient cycling technique is to visualize your foot making a perfect circle as you pedal through each full revolution. In these sessions I use a visualization exercise called "90 circles." I start by focusing fully on just my left foot for 30 revolutions, even though both feet are pedaling. I visualize that foot making 30 perfect circles. Then, when those 30 circles are complete, I focus fully on my right foot for 30 revolutions and visualize it making 30 perfect circles. Finally, for the last 30 revolutions I try to focus on both feet and visualize both feet spinning 30 perfect circles. Try this exercise several times in each High RPM Spin session.

It can be helpful to do your High RPM Spin sessions with your bike mounted on an indoor bike trainer. If you have access to a completely flat outdoor course, it won't be too difficult to maintain a constant cadence of 100-plus RPM, but a hilly course will make this session difficult and less beneficial. By putting your bike on an indoor trainer, you can ensure a constant level of resistance throughout the workout.

As we saw in Chapter 2, there is another potential advantage to doing these sessions indoors: You don't have to leave the house, so you may be able to combine these sessions in creative ways with other responsibilities. Indoor training is an effective time-management technique.

Swim Sessions

A common and major mistake is to approach swimming the same way you approach running and cycling. This is a mistake because swimming is a much different sport. Swimming is a technique sport; it has more in common with golf and tennis than it does with running and cycling.

If you have a swimming background, great! You probably already have good technique, and if so you have a great advantage. Most triathletes do not have a swimming background, however, and they are greatly limited by flawed technique. The answer for them is not to swim harder; the answer is to swim more efficiently. Most do not understand this, and they keep pounding out the laps, locking that bad form in and making it more and more difficult to correct.

My recommendation is to have an expert critique your form as soon as possible. The longer you wait, the harder it will be to make the necessary corrections. Take some one-on-one sessions with a good coach; join a Masters swim program and ask for feedback from the coach; or go to one of the great swim workshops around the country.

Because of the common misconception that swimming should be approached like running and cycling, many training for their first Iron-distance triathlon work on gradually increasing the length of their longest swim until they can swim 2.4 miles. They do this because they want to feel confident that they can finish. I recommend occasional long swims as part of your training, but only a small part (one to two times per month). The problem with a lot of long-distance swimming is that it does little to improve your technique. In fact, as you get tired your technique often deteriorates, so you end up practicing poor technique.

Let's face it, if you have the endurance to bike 112 miles and run 26.2 miles, you have the endurance to swim 2.4 miles. It is more likely that what you lack is the technique to do it efficiently. Take action and make the necessary corrections.

We will discuss proper swim technique in Chapter 11.

Rest Days

Yes, you heard me correctly. Rest days are very important. To improve your physical condition, you need to stress your body and then you need to rest it. It is during the rest periods that your body reacts to the stress, by building back stronger (discussed further in Chapter 5). If you don't rest enough to complete this build-back process, you will continually wear down, leading to injury, illness, and burnout.

In my training programs, I recommend one planned day of complete rest per week. The best place in the training schedule for the rest day is immediately after your hardest workout. I like to plan my schedule so that the training sessions become more challenging as the week goes on, and then the rest day comes just when my body really needs it.

Your work schedule may also dictate where your rest day should be. Perhaps it should fall on your busiest workday, when you have the most difficulty finding time to work out. For many who work a "normal" Monday to Friday week, Mondays work best. After your Long Bike and Long Run over the weekend, you really feel ready for some rest. Likewise, Mondays are for many people the busiest day of the week. So a rest day on Monday solves both problems.

I frequently come across athletes who do not want to take a rest day. Their work ethic commands that more is always better. I admire this work ethic, and I also understand it, because I used to approach training in much the same way. What I came to understand, however, is that sometimes more is just more, and—most importantly—sometimes more is actually less.

If you do not allow yourself enough time to recover, your great training will be wasted. The only thing you will have more of is injuries, illnesses, and mental fatigue. You will have less of what you want: conditioning and performance.

I religiously take Mondays off. In fact, I try to avoid even going into my training room on Mondays. When I come back on Tuesday, I find that I have a fresh attitude and I can't wait to dig into my training.

So far we have talked about planned rest days. There should also be room in your schedule for unplanned rest days. If you feel run down and mentally fatigued, you should take a day off. Many find this tough to do. They feel a sense of failure if they can't stick to their training plan. It's great to have a good coach in this situation, because it's hard to be objective. If you don't have a coach there to tell you to lay off and recharge your batteries, you really need to do it yourself. Remember: No one workout is going to make or break you. Don't rearrange your week. Just take one day off. Skip that day's workout. And rejoin your schedule the following day. Just forget it and go on. You will be much better off in the long run.

If you continue to feel run down, you probably need to revise your training volumes. Lower them by one third. When you feel more rested, continue to build from that point.

Listen to your body. If you are run down or feeling blah, your body is telling you to adjust your training. Make the adjustment. Your body will again tell you when it has caught up and is ready to build further.

What if an emergency comes up and you miss a day of training? Again, just skip it. One day won't make a difference in the long run. Do not try to play catch-up by doing more the next day; this is too risky. Just resume your schedule as planned.

I discuss how to adjust your schedule for missed training days further in Chapter 5.

Summary of Essential Workouts

Here again are the eight essential workouts we have discussed in this chapter:

1. The Long Run

2. The Long Ride

3. Transition Workouts

4. High Intensity Runs

5. High Intensity Rides

6. High RPM Spin Sessions

7. Swim Sessions (Technique Oriented)

8. Rest Days (sort of the non-workout workout)

These workouts are the building blocks of a highly effective Iron-distance training program. Each week of our training program will be made up of strategically placed combinations of these workouts. We will learn exactly how to do this in the next chapter, where we will discuss the Training Cycle.

IRONFIT PROFILE

Kathleen Hughes (written in 2004)
Kathleen Hughes is one of the top Masters (over 40 years of age) Ironman triathletes in the world. In 2001 Kathleen topped off an undefeated season with a victory in her age group at the most prestigious triathlon of them all, the Ironman Triathlon World Championships in Kona, Hawaii. Kathleen is married with two children and, in addition to being a super triathlete, she is a super parent, spouse, and mentor.

Kathleen raced her first triathlon in the mid-1980s when a friend encouraged her to join in. She enjoyed the fit lifestyle and the challenge of it, and kept training and racing to the point where she found herself winning a qualification slot for the World Championships in Hawaii.

Her husband Jim was supportive from the beginning. Although Jim originally assumed that the Ironman would be a onetime thing, when it became an ongoing part of Kathleen's life, he not only remained supportive, he actually became a true fan of the sport. Kathleen rates this great spousal support as her biggest asset.

Kathleen's weekdays include swimming with a Masters swim program (three days per week) between 5:30 and 7:00 a.m. Between 7:00 and 9:00 a.m., she is 100% focused on getting her two daughters off to school. From 3:00 p.m. to her 10 p.m. bedtime, Kathleen is again 100% focused on parenting responsibilities, including her daughters' activities, dinner, homework, and getting everyone ready for bed. This leaves her a training window (for everything but swimming) between 9 a.m. and 3 p.m. However, this 6-hour period is also shared with other responsibilities, such as shopping, housework, mentoring other athletes, and some volunteer activities.

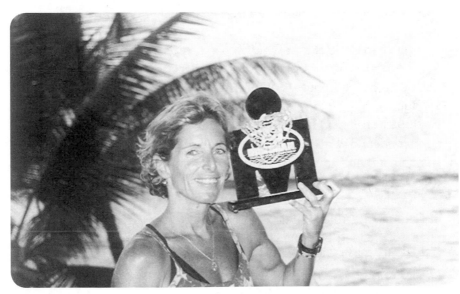

Kathleen Hughes, married, mother of two, coach . . . Iron-distance triathlete. *Photo Credit: Kathleen Hughes.*

Kathleen can usually squeeze up to 3 hours of training into this 6-hour period. This schedule of 3 hours per day, 4 days per week, plus her early morning swimming and some additional time on the weekend (when Jim is able to spend more time looking after the kids) provides Kathleen with the 20 or so hours of training a week she needs to be a world-class triathlete.

Jim has his own weekend activities as well, so planning together ahead of time is crucial to their success. In the summer Kathleen also occasionally hires a baby-sitter to open up more time for training.

Kathleen starts her day by planning out a detailed list or plan for the day. "I'm a big list writer," she says. Kathleen posts her 2-week training schedule on the kitchen door and then each day fits all of her other responsibilities onto the same list.

While Kathleen does some group training, she cautions that this is a place where time can be wasted. It can be a trade-off. If your training partners are late, it can throw off your whole schedule. When you train on your own, you don't risk being delayed by others. On the other hand, training with others can be more motivating and social. Kathleen has been lucky to find reliable training partners.

Kathleen notices that when she is busy, she tends to get more done. Because of her busy lifestyle, she needs to plan activities down to the minute, but as a result each day is far more productive.

1995 Ironman World Champion, Karen Smyers, told me that her experience was quite similar. Before she had her daughter, she sometimes had the luxury of procrastinating a bit before her training sessions, since the time pressure was not so great. Once she had her daughter, she could not afford to wait for the right moment to start her training session. As Karen put it, "Others were now relying on me."

One of Kathleen Hughes's secrets is to try to maximize her time with "Energy Givers." Kathleen describes Energy Givers as people who make you feel positive and energized when you are around them. "Energy Takers," on the other hand, are those who make you feel less energized. Kathleen believes that to take on a challenge like the Ironman, you need to be positive and keep your spirits high. Nothing can take the air out of your balloon like negative people. Kathleen tries to fill her life with positive people who give her energy. Fortunately, her immediate family is her greatest source of positive energy.

TAKE ACTION CHALLENGE: ENERGY GIVERS

Write down the names of your five greatest Energy Givers and the five worst Energy Takers. Now, after the name of each Energy Giver, make a note on how you can maintain or increase your exposure to that person. Then write a note after the name of each Energy Taker on how you can decrease or eliminate your time with that person.

CHAPTER 4

The Training Cycle

"Life shrinks and expands in proportion
to one's courage."

—Anais Nin

What if I told you there is a way to train in which the total benefit of your training can be greater than the sum of its parts? If you are a busy person, trying to squeeze out precious training time, I bet you would be interested. Well, guess what? There is, and it's through the effective use of training cycles.

The importance of training cycles is both overlooked and misunderstood by most athletes. But for those who embrace them, the result is truly synergistic training.

I find that most busy athletes will discover at least some of the Essential Workouts described in Chapter 3 through magazines, books, and other training resources. They then go about deciding when to schedule these key sessions in their training week.

They may schedule some based on the group training opportunities available to them. For example, the local running club may have a regularly scheduled track workout on Wednesday evenings, so that's when they do their High Intensity running intervals. Or the bike shop has a weekly group ride, or the YMCA has a regularly scheduled swim. Whatever is not covered by these group workouts is then just randomly squeezed into the remaining available days of the week.

The potential problem with this approach is that a randomly grouped bunch of workouts probably do not add up to an effective training program. What you do on Monday will affect your body on Tuesday and probably even Wednesday. What you do on Tuesday will affect your body on Wednesday

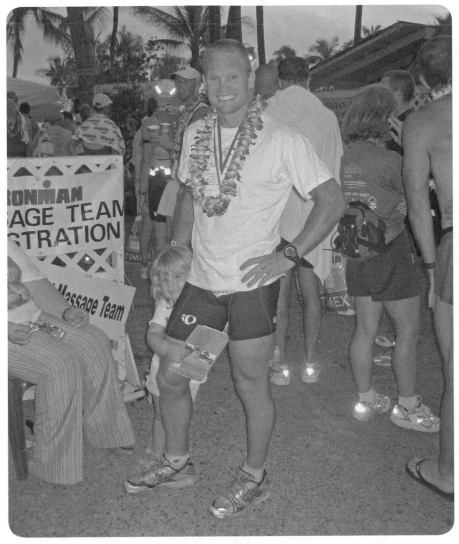

Nick Horton, married, father, business executive . . . Iron-distance triathlete.
Photo Credit: Anna Horton.

and probably even Thursday, and so on. A training day does not stand alone. It is part of a delicate, interlocking chain—the weekly training cycle.

As we will see in Chapter 5, we do not improve fitness merely by stressing the body. We grow strong by stressing the body in a very specific way, and then resting it and allowing it to adapt. Those who randomly pack together their workouts may easily violate this principle and thereby diminish or negate the training benefit of yesterday's workout, today's workout, and possibly tomorrow's.

What if you could select just the right workout for today, one that would not only yield a specific training benefit, but would also prepare your body for what you plan to do tomorrow? And what if tomorrow your selected workout (1) not only allowed your body to further absorb today's workout, but (2) also derived another specific training benefit and (3) prepared your body for the following day's work?

Now this would be highly effective training! The kind of training we talked about above, in which the total benefit is greater than the sum of its parts. This is exactly what an effective training plan does. And it's not only limited to the short-term outlook of this week. Today's workout should provide a training benefit, and it should set up tomorrow's workout. This week should provide a training benefit, and it should set up next week. And yes, this month should provide a training benefit, and it should set us up for a training benefit next month.

Short-Term Weekly Training Cycles

Most athletes make the mistake of training pretty much the same way all the time. They do the same swim workouts whenever they go to the pool. They participate in the same weekly group ride, where they always start out at an easy, social pace and then pick it up and ride hard at the end. They run the same favorite course from their house, usually at about the same pace. And so on, and so on.

I remember a favorite saying from my business career: "The definition of insanity is doing the same thing over and over, and expecting a different outcome." Unfortunately, this is exactly how most athletes approach their training.

While we do want to establish a weekly pattern of training, so we know roughly what activity we will do each day, the exact details of each regularly scheduled training session should vary from week to week. It's useful to have a weekly pattern; it makes our week predictable for scheduling and time management purposes. But the individual workouts within the weekly pattern need to change continually.

While it's not necessary to master every concept that goes into designing an effective weekly cycle, as they are built into the actual IronFit training programs presented in Chapter 7, let's take a look at three of the most important ones.

● Alternate High Intensity Days with Low Intensity Days

The effects of a High Intensity run or bike session can take over 24 hours to recover from, sometimes 48 hours or more. The important fact to remember is that recovery is essential to the training process. A specific workout stresses the body in a specific way. It's the body's natural reaction to try to grow stronger opposite that stress. To make sure this happens, we need to follow the stress with the proper period of rest. We stress it, and then we must rest it.

If you stress your body with a High Intensity run today, it is likely that another High Intensity run tomorrow will not allow this process of growing stronger to occur; in fact, it may even break the body down by overstressing it. Overstressing not only negates the potential benefit of our hard training, it also risks injury and setback as well.

A better choice for the day after a High Intensity run is a lower intensity session, for example an easy run or bike, or a low intensity Transition Session. These types of sessions are more likely to allow recovery and the absorption of the High Intensity run's training benefit, while also focusing on another training element.

Furthermore, having had a low intensity session today, we may be ready for another High Intensity session tomorrow, perhaps this time a bike session.

The training programs in Chapter 7 will show you how to integrate High Intensity sessions properly with other workouts.

● Surprise the Body

As we said, many athletes tend to do the same exact workouts in the same way, over and over. They run the same courses at roughly the same paces. They pick up the pace at about the same time.

The problem with getting trapped in a routine is that we are no longer stimulating the body to grow in some way. The body has become so accustomed to doing the exact same thing that it no longer responds with fitness gains. Furthermore, the body becomes well-trained to do those specific workouts, but not as well-trained to react to the dynamic conditions of actual racing.

We need to continually "surprise" the body with slightly different, and often increased, challenges in training. We want to introduce small, incremental changes in each workout to stimulate continued growth.

For example, we may do a recurring session Fridays in which a High Intensity run occurs within a longer run performed at a comfortable, aerobic pace. The amount of High Intensity running will vary from one week to the next, as will the total length of the run. In each session we will challenge our bodies in slightly different ways, thereby providing the stimulus for them to grow and become fitter. For example, take these three workouts. Z2 indicates a moderate, aerobic pace, and Z4 indicates a fast, anaerobic pace (these terms will be explained later).

Week 1: Friday run: 45 minute Z2 (at 30 minutes, insert 5 minutes Z4)

Week 2: Friday run: 45 minute Z2 (at 30 minutes, insert 7.5 minute Z4)

Week 3: Friday run: 60 minute Z2 (at 45 minutes, insert 7.5 minute Z4)

This is a regularly scheduled session that varies slightly from week to week. In this example, it's always a run and it always contains a High Intensity portion, but the variables change modestly from one week to the next. In the second week, the body is "surprised" by a longer High Intensity portion. In the third week, the body is surprised by a longer overall duration, and the Higher Intensity portion begins at a different point in the run. Each change is incremental and, in this case, more challenging.

● **Proper Single-Sport Spacing**

Best results are also achieved when we spread out across the week our sessions in each sport. As an extreme example: Swimming Monday and Tuesday, cycling Wednesday and Thursday, and running Friday and Saturday is not an efficient way to train. While we don't want to do every sport every day, we do want to keep our sport-specific muscles active throughout the week.

As a general guideline, you don't want more than 3 days to pass without doing a particular sport. This will help to keep sport-specific muscles engaged and make continued progress possible. This is particularly important in a highly technique-oriented sport like swimming, where your form will deteriorate if it is not frequently reinforced.

The three concepts discussed above—alternating high and low intensity days, surprising the body, and single-sport spacing—are among the most important guiding principles for building an efficient weekly training cycle. The key point to remember is that an effective weekly training cycle is not a random grouping of the Essential Workouts. Our training benefit is maximized when we strategically place these workouts within the week, subject to whatever restrictions life throws in the way.

Long-Term Training Cycles

As discussed above, not only is each training day related to the days before and after it, so are the weeks and months.

Just as we can benefit from incremental training changes from day to day, and incremental training progression from week to week, we can also benefit most by approaching our entire training year in much the same way. The concept of benefiting from interrelated training phases over a longer period of time is commonly referred to as "periodization."

Ideally, we want our training to progress through a planned series of cycles over a long period, and to bring us to a peak level of conditioning at just the right time to maximize our performance. This is particularly important in Iron-distance training, where it all comes down to one big day.

I have had success with hundreds of Iron-distance triathletes using a periodization approach based on the following four training phases:

- "Base" Training Phase

- "Build" Training Phase

- "Peak" Training Phase

- Recovery/Maintenance Training Phase

All three IronFit training programs in Chapter 7 follow this periodization formula.

Following is a detailed discussion of the Base Training Phase, the Build Training Phase, and the Peak Training Phase. I cover the Recovery/Maintenance Phase separately in Chapter 19.

Base Training Phase

The initial 10-week IronFit Base Training Phase focuses on (1) acclimating the athlete to triathlon training, (2) establishing and building an aerobic base, and (3) building sport-specific technique.

This is one of my favorite phases because I love aerobic training. We will discuss aerobic training in detail in Chapter 6, but for our purposes at this point, we are talking about low to moderate intensity training. Simply put, training at a comfortable level of exertion.

If done consistently, aerobic training makes you feel great. Your body gradually becomes fitter, leaner, and faster, and learns how to burn fat more efficiently as fuel, which it will need to do to go the Iron-distance. You don't have to get mentally fired up for these workouts. In fact, this can be the most social time of the year. Find some training partners with a similar aerobic pace (and related heart rate zone), and just go out and enjoy these runs and rides. Chapter 6 will explain how to calculate your proper heart rate training zones.

Think, "Time in the zone." That's what I tell the athletes I coach. This training phase is mostly about keeping your heart rate within the proper range (zone), and then just putting in the time. Your body will respond. Six-time Ironman World Champion Mark Allen refers to this as the "patience phase." You want to be patient and resist the temptation to go faster.

The fact that this phase is relatively easy and enjoyable does not imply that it is unimportant. The Base Phase is very important, possibly the most important to your eventual success in your Iron-distance triathlon. The foundation you establish here is essential. It prepares you for all of the longer duration and higher intensity training that lies ahead.

Many athletes skip or minimize this phase, hoping to catch up later. The problem is, you can't make this up. It can't be faked in Iron-distance. Skipping the Base Phase is like building a house without a foundation. The house will crumble when conditions become difficult.

We also want to focus on technique during the Base Phase. Use this time to fine-tune your form as much as possible, before you get to the longer and higher intensity sessions ahead. We want to build on efficient technique. We increase our ultimate potential by improving technique.

As we've seen, this is particularly true of swimming. If your form is inefficient, no matter how much work you do, you are limiting your speed potential. For most triathletes, swimming endurance is not the problem; they are already extremely fit. The challenge is technique. The Base Phase is the best time to improve this aspect. Technique will be discussed in greater detail in Chapter 11.

● Build Training Phase

In the 10-week Build Phase we prepare ourselves to take on the challenging training of the final Peak Phase. In the Build Phase, we continue to increase the duration of our training sessions, we introduce High Intensity sessions, and our training becomes more race specific, including actually competing in our first practice race, an Olympic distance triathlon (1.5K swim, 40K bike, and 10K run).

These more challenging training elements are introduced and increased gradually. The concept of gradual adaptation will be discussed in detail in the next chapter, but at this point it is important to understand that our bodies will only adapt well to changes in training if they are introduced at the proper rate.

If we increase the duration or intensity of workouts too quickly, the body is likely to break down and suffer injury and setback. If we introduce these changes too slowly, our fitness level may not sufficiently improve, because the stimuli were not great enough. As will be explained in Chapter 5, the key to becoming fitter is increasing the duration and intensity of training at the proper rate. As a general guideline, we want to avoid week-to-week increases in duration of more than 10% in our combined training.

How much High Intensity training is appropriate in the Build Phase? In general, most athletes training for the Iron-distance do too much High Intensity work. High Intensity training should be limited to a maximum of only 10% of the total combined cycling and running durations. I will discuss High Intensity training further in Chapter 6.

• Peak Training Phase

This final 10-week training phase is the most exciting and challenging part of the IronFit training cycle. It starts with a final dress rehearsal: a Half Iron-distance practice race (1.2-mile swim, 56-mile bike, and 13.1-mile run). This is an opportunity to test ourselves and see how we perform in actual race conditions. It is also an opportunity to identify any areas of weakness that need attention over the final weeks.

Following the practice race, we will increase training durations and intensities for about 5 weeks (depending on the training program) until they reach their peak 3 weeks before the actual race date. This is crunch time. Here we will do our most challenging and time-consuming training. This is also when all of the time-management techniques we will discuss come into play.

Finally, we enter a 3-week "taper." During the taper we gradually bring down both the duration and intensity of training, right up to race day. Done properly, tapering will bring us to the starting line rested and energized, yet without having lost any fitness. Hitting a perfect peak is difficult, but that is exactly what the training plans in Chapter 7 are designed to do. We want to time it perfectly and arrive at our absolute best on race day. Super-fit, well-rested, and mentally ready for a great race experience.

The 10-week Peak Phase can be segmented as follows:

- **Weeks 1–2:** 1 challenging week of training, followed by a mini 1-week taper and then our final dress rehearsal, a Half Iron-distance competition.

- **Weeks 3–7:** Gradually increasing both duration of training and High Intensity portions to peak levels.

- **Weeks 8–10:** A crisp 3-week taper with a gradual decrease in durations and High Intensity portions. Concluding with our big day, the Iron-distance triathlon.

Chapter 7 will present three complete 30-week IronFit training programs, all of which will incorporate the short- and long-term training cycle concepts presented in this chapter. But before we get to the training programs, let's address this Take Action Challenge.

TAKE ACTION CHALLENGE: "MARK YOUR CALENDAR"

Let's not just talk the talk—let's walk the walk!

Select an Ironman race you think you may be interested in signing up for. Mark the race on your calendar right now. Then, working backward, fill in all of the above dates: the date the 10-week Base Phase begins, the date the 10-week Build Phase begins, and the date the 10-week Peak Phase begins.

It's fine to think about training cycles in the abstract, but in my experience it's far better to choose a real race date, get out a calendar or training log, and actually write in the training phases. By doing this you actually see which months of the year each phase will fall into, given a particular race day. Then you can compare the training calendar with your work schedule and family obligations and really get a clear sense of what issues, if any, need to be worked out to make the dream a reality.

So do it now! Whether you are already entered in a race or whether you have a race in mind, get out your calendar and plot out the key dates in the training cycle. There is real power in writing it down—in making the commitment. Take yourself through this analysis. It will help put you on the path to achieving your dream.

To help you get started, here's an example. Suppose an athlete chooses to enter the 2012 Ironman Florida, which may be scheduled for November 3.
The phases would fall like this:

Base Phase: *April 9 through June 17*

Build Phase: *June 18 through August 26 (first practice race, the Olympic distance, around July 9)*

Peak Phase: *August 27 through November 3 (second practice race, Half Iron-distance, around September 9; peak volumes reached September 10 to October 15)*

Race day: *November 3*

IRONFIT PROFILE

Jan Wanklyn (written in 2004)

Australian Pro Jan Wanklyn has been one of the most consistent top Iron-distance performers. She has completed 29 races over the last 20 years, and has three overall victories at Ironman New Zealand, as well as overall championships at Ironman Australia and Ironman Europe. Amazingly Jan took a couple of years off around the birth of her daughter Reanin, and then came back to pick up just where she left off, with victories at Ironman New Zealand and the Philadelphia Marathon.

In addition to being a parent and a pro triathlete, Jan has her own massage/performance care business. She combines massage, Active Release Therapy, and other state-of-the-art techniques to help athletes and regular people stay in top health and perform at their best. In addition to working with her own clients, Jan is an ART instructor and helps others to learn and develop their skills. Jan also continues to attend frequent training programs herself, as she is always looking to build her skills as well.

Finally, Jan mentors other athletes, some formally and some informally, on training, racing, and nutrition. Her guidance is highly sought after and well-respected in the triathlon world.

Champion endurance athlete, full-time parent, successful business owner, mentor for other athletes; how does she make it all work?

Like many of the Iron-distance triathletes I have talked about, Jan Wanklyn is a master at time management. Jan and her pro triathlete husband Ken Glah are well-organized and plan out their schedules together like a well-oiled machine. Jan employs virtually all of the "Big Five" time-management tips I presented in Chapter 2, plus adds plenty of her own.

Following are some of Jan Wanklyn's best time-management secrets:

1. **Early Bird Training:** "I always need to work out in the morning, so that I can set up my appointments for the afternoon and evening. This can be tough after a long training day, but it adds to the challenge of it all."

2. **Participating in a Masters Swimming Program:** "I do an early morning swim Masters, which is the least disruptive for the family. They don't even know I am gone. Usually I run as well. Then home to get Reanin to school and then possibly a bike ride, depending on the day."

3. **Sharing Parental Responsibilities:** "Ken and I work around each other's schedules and he is the main transport/taxi for our daughter as his work schedule is less rigid than mine." (In addition to being a pro triathlete, husband Ken owns a sports travel business.) "We have always shared responsibilities with Reanin and the house. We do what we are efficient and good at; sometimes there is overlap, but not often."

4. **Long Training Sessions during the Week:** Whereas most athletes need to schedule their longer training sessions for the weekend, when they have more time available, Jan is able to schedule them for during the week due to the nature of her business. This is a big advantage as it allows her to enjoy more activities with her daughter on the weekend.

5. **Being Flexible Mentally:** "I try to be flexible when things don't work out as planned, because it's all planned down to a science. If you hit one red light that wasn't accounted for, you may have to cut the day's workout short, and that's OK. In the scheme of things, it really doesn't matter. Once we had Reanin, it was more the challenge of being able to get most of it in and being organized to do it, and getting to the starting line healthy and fit, than actual race day performance. The emphasis changes as there is greater balance for you as an athlete."

6. **Indoor Training:** "I do much indoor riding now, so I can be here when Reanin wakes and Ken is out. I can get a better workout indoors. Reanin would come down and watch television while we bike, or we would set up her bike with the Computrainer."

7. **Finding Ways to Include Daughter:** "Reanin has come to many track workouts and been in charge of the watch for timing, or she's played in the long jump sand pit or even done some running on the track. She'll also bring a friend to the pool so she is occupied while we work out. This has been an option and an easy way to make it work for us."

8. **Combining Races with Vacation:** "Ken and I decided early on that we could not do the same Ironman races . . . too much stress on us all. We all go to Hawaii and that is a vacation for our daughter . . . not us. She gets to go to many places when we race and has a vacation, as we never do the summer vacation thing. Way too many people and it is our big training time for triathlons."

CHAPTER 5

The Principle of Gradual Adaptation

"You are your own creation and you are
what you believe yourself to be."

—*Cory Everson*

The principle of "gradual adaptation" asserts that we can achieve our desired fitness by applying the proper training stimuli at the appropriate rate. This principle guides my approach to training, since my philosophy is that we need to work with our bodies, not against them, to achieve the best results. You will find the principle of gradual adaptation built into all three of the 30-week IronFit training programs presented in Chapter 7.

It's not surprising many people drawn to the Iron-distance challenge are highly accomplished and driven people. These are typically not the kind of personalities to avoid obstacles. More likely, they have been successful by attacking obstacles and overcoming them through hard work and perseverance.

These are wonderful qualities but sometimes they are applied incorrectly to training. I understand this mind-set because I used to approach my training in much the same way. I viewed any obstacles that arose as the enemy, and I worked to "defeat" them.

When my body sent pain signals, I didn't see them as helpful messages; I saw them as something to be overcome. I relied on strength of mind to override what my body was telling me. I believed in the old "no pain, no gain" philosophy. My mind was going to force my body into shape, no matter how much it complained.

This was a big mistake. The pain signals often developed into injuries, and then into major setbacks. Mentally I ended up discouraged and frustrated. Clearly, no one was winning the mind-versus-body battle.

I now know better. I understand that the mind and body must be partners in training. Those "pain signals" contain information. They are providing us with early warning signs to help us make intelligent training decisions. By training intelligently, we can remain free of injury and improve our fitness consistently, year after year, without setbacks.

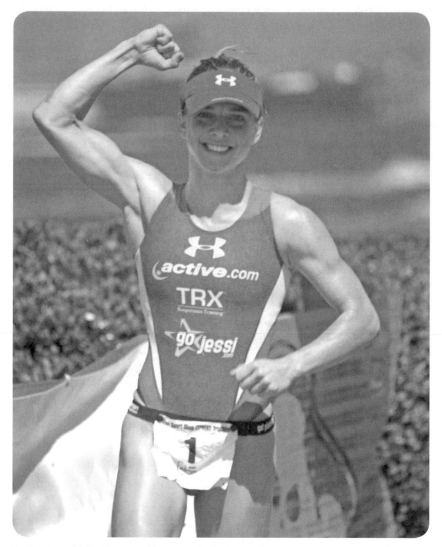

Professional triathlete and Ironman Baja 70.3 Champion Jessi Stensland. *Photo Credit: DeSanti Photography.*

The wonderful news is this: Our bodies are able to adapt and change in many ways and to a much greater extent than many of us realize. The secret is to work with your body, and at your body's own rate of adaptation.

The concept of gradual adaptation is particularly important for those just starting out, and those who have been away from training for some time. If you go out on the first day of your new program and swim for 1 hour, cycle for 2 hours, run for 1 hour, and then finish up with some strength training, you will probably end up so badly injured that you won't be able to train again for months. Be patient. Accept the concept of gradual adaptation and gradually ease into training. Work with your body's natural rate of absorbing training.

Before we begin our discussion, some key definitions:

- **Duration:** The length of a training session as measured by time, not by distance.

- **Intensity:** The level of effort as measured by heart rate. For example, aerobic training takes place at a moderate intensity, while anaerobic training takes place at a high intensity.

- **Frequency:** The number of training sessions over a given period of time; for example, three running sessions per week.

- **Volume:** The combination of duration, intensity, and frequency. In other words, total training volume increases with an increase to any one of these variables, or any combination of them.

If you increase training volume too much, your body will not be able to adapt and some kind of breakdown is likely. This could be an injury, an illness, or just mental burnout. On the other hand, if you increase training volume too little, it may not be sufficient to stimulate change, and the desired training benefit will not be obtained.

What you want is to find just the right changes in duration, intensity, and frequency to effect the desired results. You want to work with your body's natural rate of training absorption.

We are all different, of course, and what works for one athlete may not work for another. There are some general guidelines, however, that tend to work for the vast majority of athletes.

I have found the "10% rule" generally applies in most situations. Namely, increases in total weekly duration should be limited to no more than 10% from one week to the next. While there are plenty of exceptions to this, and it's really more of a guideline than a rule, the 10% rule is a good place to start.

We will begin our discussion by considering some practical applications.

Increases in Duration

Let's take the example of an individual whose exercise regimen over the last few months has been to run 30 minutes at a comfortable pace, three times a week (i.e., total weekly training equals 90 minutes). What if, in an effort to increase his level of fitness, this athlete changed his program to running 1 hour at a comfortable pace, three times a week?

Intensity (comfortable pace) and frequency (three times per week) have remained the same, but duration has increased 100%. Our training volume has therefore significantly increased. For the vast majority of athletes, this extreme increase in duration would lead to injury or some other form of setback.

Now, with the concept of gradual adaptation in mind, let's instead increase duration by 10% per week for several weeks.

WEEK	TRAINING PER WEEK (MINUTES)
0	90
1	99
2	109
3	120
4	133
5	145
6	160
7	175

In the chart above, the athlete increases his duration by 10% per week, and is able to more than double his weekly training duration in just over 7 weeks. This athlete is far more likely to achieve his desired fitness goal—doubled duration. He will avoid the frustration of a setback and gain confidence and enthusiasm from his success. After the same 7 weeks, the athlete in the first example may just be getting over an injury, about to start all over again.

● Reducing Duration Every Fourth Week

In the above example, we increase durations by 10% each week, for 7 straight weeks. While this was presented this way to illustrate a point and to keep the example simple, I would not usually suggest increasing durations for 7 weeks straight. For many athletes, I have found that a 4-week duration "drop off" approach works best in the long run. By increasing durations for 3 straight weeks, but then reducing durations (usually by 5 to 20%) in the fourth week, the athlete better absorbs the benefits of their training, rejuvenates them-selves, and becomes more resistant to stagnation or injury.

This can lead to an acceptable exception to the 10% rule. Following the "drop-off" week, durations can be increased by as much as 25%, as long as the average increase for the 4-week period is 10% or less.

Increases in Intensity

The 10% rule also applies to intensity; however, what increases gradually is the percentage of High Intensity training relative to total training.

For example, take the same athlete who has been running 30 minutes at a comfortable pace, three times a week. In an effort to increase his level of fitness, this athlete decides to change his program by including an 18-minute High Intensity (race pace) effort, inserted in the middle of one of his three weekly runs.

Duration (90 minutes per week) and frequency (three times per week) remain the same, but the High Intensity portion has increased from zero to 18 minutes (20% of the weekly total). Training volume has therefore significantly increased.

For the vast majority of athletes, this extreme increase in intensity would risk injury or some other setback.

Now, with the concept of gradual adaptation in mind, let's instead increase the High Intensity portion gradually over time. We will start with a 4.5-minute High Intensity portion in the weekly run, and then increase it gradually over several weeks.

WEEK	MINUTES OF HIGH INTENSITY	% OF HIGH INTENSITY
0	0	0
1	4.5	5
2	9.0	10
3	13.5	15
4	18.0	20

In this example, the athlete increases his High Intensity portion to 18 minutes in only 4 weeks, but accomplishes this by gradually increasing this portion by 4.5 minutes per week (or by increments of only 5% of the total duration). With this gradual approach, it is far more likely that the athlete's body will be able to grow stronger and adapt to these changes, without injury or setback.

Increases in Frequency

The 10% rule doesn't apply directly to frequency. However, it does apply indirectly, as increases in frequency will impact weekly duration.

For example, take an athlete who runs three times per week for 30 minutes, for a total of 90 minutes of training. She can add a fourth run per week, but if she keeps all four of these runs at 30 minutes, her total weekly duration will increase from 90 to 120 minutes. This would be an increase of 33%—a clear violation of the 10% rule.

The best way to accomplish the objective of adding the fourth run is to shorten some of the runs to keep the increase in weekly duration within the 10% rule; then the runs can be gradually increased as desired. For instance:

WEEK	DURATION OF RUNS (MINUTES)	TOTAL DURATION (MINUTES)	% INCREASE
0	30+30+30	90	0
1	25+25+25+24	99	10
2	30+25+30+24	109	10
3	30+30+30+30	120	10

In this example, the athlete adds a fourth run, but decreases the length of each run to stay within the 10% rule. Then she increases the lengths of the individual runs each week, while continuing to limit the total increase to 10%. Within only 3 weeks, the fourth run has been added, and all runs are at the original length of 30 minutes. By taking this approach, it is far more likely that the athlete will be able to adapt successfully to the desired increase without injury or setback.

Adjusting for Missed Workouts

Not only do we need to apply the concept of gradual adaptation in designing our training program, but we also need to apply it when making adjustments for unforeseen training interruptions.

What if you miss a period of training due to an illness, a business trip, or some other reason? After not training for several days, do you just jump back into your program where you left off, or will this violate the concept of gradual adaptation?

First of all, you should not train if you are ill. Health comes before fitness. You should always seek proper medical care for any illness, and you should not resume training until a qualified medical professional has determined that you are ready to do so.

Over the years, I have seen many athletes try to train through illness, and it was always a bad idea. Instead of just taking a few days off to get better, they ended up aggravating and greatly prolonging their illness. Instead of losing a few days they often lost or compromised weeks of training. So listen to your body and do the right thing.

Following are some guidelines on how to adjust your training for missed workouts.

- **1 day missed:** If you miss 1 day of training, for any reason, just skip it. Missing one workout is never going to matter in the long run, and it is risky to try to catch up by doubling up workouts.

- **2–3 days missed:** Skip the lost days and rejoin your normal training program, but on the first day back only do half of the scheduled training. Resume full training on the second day back.

- **4–6 days missed:** Rejoin your training program (again, skip the missed days), but when you rejoin your program, do one-third of the scheduled training on the first 2 days back, and two-thirds of the scheduled training on the next 2 days back. Resume full training on the fifth day back.

- **7 or more days missed:** Possibly reconsider the timing of your goal and redesign your training program accordingly.

Keep in mind that the above guidelines are all subject to the 10% rule. In others words, apply the guideline, but then also apply the 10% rule to the entire training schedule to see if any further adjustment is necessary. The next training week's duration (the week after the comeback week) should not be increased by more than 10% over the average of the past 3 weeks.

Let's consider an example. You are called out on a business trip on short notice, and you are not able to complete about half of your planned workouts. Your total weekly training duration slips from 9 hours the previous 3 weeks to only 5 hours during the week of the trip. Your schedule had actually called for you to increase to 10 hours during the business trip week and 11 hours the following week.

How should you adjust your training for the week following the business trip? Some possible options:

1. Ignore the fact that you went from a 9-hour week to a 5-hour week, and rejoin your schedule as is with an 11-hour week.

2. Make up for the 5 hours missed during your business trip week by adding them to the planned 11-hour week, making it a 16-hour week. This is a favorite solution with type A triathletes!

3. Do a 5.5-hour training week, because 5 hours plus 10% is 5.5 hours.

4. Revise your training duration for next week, limiting it to no more than 10% more than the average of the preceding 4 weeks.

Let's review these options:

1. You may be able to get away with this option once or twice a season, but it is not recommended. The risk of injury and setback is too great.

2. This is the probably the worst choice. It violates the gradual adaptation principle and is highly risky. Athletes do this because they feel guilty for missing training; only a complete catch-up will set their minds at ease.

3. This is probably being overly cautious. If you have been training consistently over time, this will not be necessary.

4. This is usually the best choice. If you have been training consistently for at least a couple of months, apply the 10% rule to your average duration over the past 4 weeks.

Following is the calculation:

Add up total hours of the past 4 weeks: 9 + 9 + 9 + 5 = 32 hours.

Find the average: 32 hours/4 = 8.0 hours.

Increase the average by 10%: 8.0 hours + 10% = 8.8 hours.

Therefore, the next week's training should be adjusted from 11 hours to 8.8 hours.

Summary

Gradual adaptation is one of the most important training principles. It requires patience and discipline to embrace the principle, but if you do you will enjoy significant improvements in your training and greatly increase your chances of achieving your Ironman goal.

While it is important to understand gradual adaptation, the three 30-week training programs presented in Chapter 7 are all built around this principle. These training programs, with occasional adjustments, will keep you on the road to the Ironman.

AN IRONFIT MOMENT

1% Improvements

The following was written by the author in early 1999.

As I stood on the edge of the crashing surf, I thought to myself, "This is going to be the race." After three years of middle-of-the-pack performances, I planned to place in the top three in my age group. With butterflies in my stomach and a lump in my throat, I thought, "Today I will finally make a trip to the podium."

Well, that was the plan anyway. I know it sounds silly. It's not that big a deal—to hear your name announced and go up to receive some tacky award. But I wanted to experience it. Even if it was just that once. After all, nobody gets into triathlon for acclaim. I liked the sport. I enjoyed the lifestyle. I loved the excitement of showing up at a race early Sunday morning and giving it my all. After three years and over twenty races, however, it would sure be nice to crack the top three.

I picked a local short-course race held each year at the Jersey Shore. After training harder than I had ever trained before, I walked down to the edge of the surf that morning prepared to give it everything I had.

Eighth place in my age group. Ugh! "Well, that's OK," I thought. I wasn't really that disappointed. I did show some improvement and I did finish in the top ten. "After all," I thought, "I race triathlon because I enjoy it."

A few weeks passed and when I came home from work one day, I grabbed the mail and sat down at the kitchen table to read the race results. I found my name in eighth place in my age group and then skimmed up to the time of the third-place finisher. Something struck me. While this competitor was five places ahead of me, his time was only 1 minute and 40 seconds faster. I quickly did the math. To my surprise, I discovered that his time was only 1% faster than mine. Only 1%! It hit me like a revelation. I remember asking myself, "Can I get 1% faster?" I thought for a few seconds and then answered, "Yes, of course I can!"

Ideas started popping into my head: Join a Masters swim program . . . attend a cycling clinic . . . find a new running coach. I started writing them down. Start a strength training program . . . find a good book on nutrition . . . work on my hill-climbing technique. The ideas kept coming faster and faster. Suddenly, I realized that even after three years in the sport, I had really only scratched the surface. There were so many ways to become 1% faster that I could go on listing them for hours.

Occasionally I would dream about winning my age group at the world championship in Hawaii. It was fun but it really only reminded me of how ridiculously far away that ultimate dream was. On the other hand, focusing on how I could achieve a "1% improvement" was highly motivating. It was very achievable. When you are down in the valley, the mountain peak seems impossibly high. The best thing to do is to forget about the peak and to focus completely on the very next step in the climb.

Since stumbling onto the concept of 1% improvements many years ago, I have used it time after time to stay focused and motivated. Once I have achieved a 1% improvement, then—and only then—I focus on where to find my next 1% improvement. Each time I have asked myself the question, "Can I become 1% faster?" I have never had a shortage of ideas. I also came to realize that the concept of "1% improvements" is not limited to athletics. All success begins with the first "1% improvement." Ask yourself right now, Can I perform 1% better at my job? Can I be a 1% better husband or wife? Can I be a 1% better person? If your answer is "yes" to any of these questions—and it surely is—write down a list of all the ways you can think of to achieve a 1% improvement. Then pick a couple of items from your list and go to work on them. Take action.

This past February, many years and races after I first discovered the concept of "1% improvements," I received the final results in the mail from the 1998 Hawaii Ironman World Championships. Like so many times before, I sat at the kitchen table, flipping through the results when I came across my name. I looked with pride, remembering the second-place finish in my age group. It was my best finish ever, but still I fantasized for a moment about how wonderful it would be to win my age group. To win the big one. I looked at the winner's time and subtracted my own. It was a little over five minutes. I did the math, and guess what? It was just about 1%. As I reached for a pad and pencil, I asked myself, "Can I get 1% faster?"

IRONFIT PROFILE

Andrew Jones (written in 2004)

Andrew Jones works for Lehman Brothers, a major investment-banking firm in New York City. He commutes to his job each day by train from his home in suburban New Jersey. His total door-to-door weekday time is between 11 and 12 hours. He is thirty-five years old. He and his wife of thirteen years have two daughters, ages three years and ten months. Andrew, who is British, came to New York with his family on a work assignment with his company. In addition, Andrew also travels a great deal, both on business and to visit family.

Andrew became an Ironman in July 2001 at Ironman USA in Lake Placid, New York. His journey to the Ironman did not happen overnight. He started out running road races and then marathons several years before. He eventually tried short-course triathlon and then attempted the Half Iron-distance in 2000 at the Gulf Coast Triathlon in May and at the Blackwater Eagleman Triathlon in June. His success at the Half Iron-distance, combined with the fact that his brother, Adrian, completed an Iron-distance race back in Great Britain, led him to take on the Ironman.

Andrew is not outspoken about his triathlon dreams at work. He wants to maintain balance in his life and worries that some might question his dedication to his work, and think his hobby too extreme.

So here we have someone with a demanding career in the financial capital of the world, a significant commute each day, a wife and two young children, and the dream to do the Ironman. How does he do it? How can he possibly accomplish all of these goals?

Andrew is extremely organized and manages his days down to the small increments of time. Andrew often gets up early to get a swim in at the local pool, eats breakfast with his oldest daughter, and then catches the train to work. Here we see how Andrew touches on all three major areas of his life, athletics, family, and career, within a very short period of time.

In addition to the "Big Five" time-management techniques discussed earlier, Andrew uses these methods:

- **Three Daily Opportunities to Train:** He sees each weekday as having three opportunities to train: before work, at lunchtime, and in the evening. Morning is the preferred time, lunchtime is the second choice, and evening is the last chance. He attempts to schedule his training for early morning; if something comes up, he lets it slide into the second or third time slots.

- **Do Two Things at Once:** Andrew sometimes sets up his indoor trainer in his baby's room, so he can spend time with his daughter while he gets his training in.

- **Run or Cycle There:** Andrew looks for opportunities throughout the day to combine his training with other responsibilities. For example, Andrew may not drive with his family to the pool for a weekend family swim, he may choose to run or cycle over to meet them there.

- **Helpful Relatives:** He invites his mother-in-law and other relatives to visit frequently, as this provides a helpful and trusted baby-sitter.

- **Achieve Balance:** Andrew always tries to achieve balance among his priorities, and he views the challenge from that perspective.

CHAPTER 6

Effective Heart Rate Training

"Those who dance are considered to be
insane by those who can't hear the music."

—*George Carlin*

There is no "magic bullet" in Iron-distance training, but heart rate training comes close. Effective heart rate training is the best way to maximize your training benefit and minimize your training time.

There are so many books written about heart rate training, and you see so many athletes out training with their heart rate monitors on, you would think this was a training principle the vast majority of athletes have nailed down. Well, guess what? They haven't.

Having worked with hundreds of athletes over the years, I have found that most athletes train in the wrong heart rate zones most of the time. Considering all of the attention given to this topic, I know this is difficult to believe.

These athletes are therefore training inefficiently, wasting their precious training time with "junk miles," and achieving far less than optimal training benefits. With a career and important family responsibilities, who has time for "junk miles?" Every minute of training time needs to count.

The good news is that even experienced triathletes can achieve significant performance improvements through more effective heart rate training. I have found that even athletes who have competed in triathlon for many years will achieve significant performance gains just by correcting this one element. I have coached triathletes with over 15 years of experience who have taken over an hour off their best Iron-distance times after making adjustments to get them into the proper training zones.

One great example of this is veteran triathlete Ray Campeau. In his 40s and after 20 years of triathlon racing, Ray had not gone below an 11:15 for

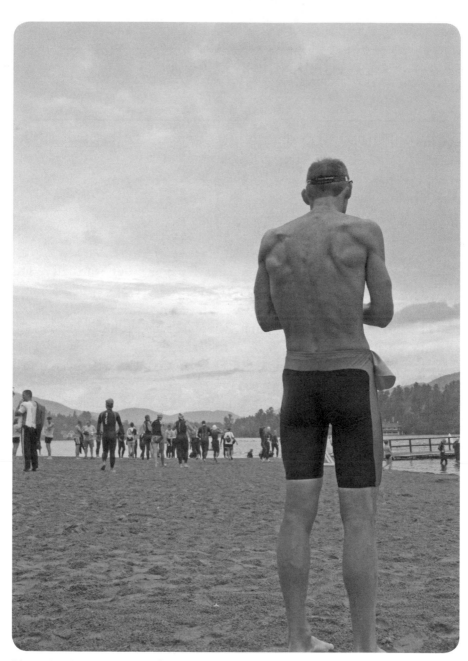

Photo Credit: Lynn Kellogg/www.trilifephotos.com.

an Iron-distance triathlon. After working with my IronFit training approach for less than a year, Ray not only raced to a time of 10:12 at Ironman USA (Lake Placid, N.Y.), one of the most challenging courses, but in doing so, qualified for the Ironman World Championships in Hawaii.

If you follow the 30-week training programs presented in Chapter 7, you will be investing your training time in just the right heart rate zones and for just the right proportion of time. At the end of this chapter, we will calculate your personal heart rate zones, to be used in these training plans. With the right heart rate zones and the right training program, you will achieve your Iron-distance goal.

As I have said before, one thing we are not going to do in this book is present a bunch of complicated scientific and technical lingo. I am going to tell you exactly what you need to do to train intelligently and efficiently. With that in mind, the following section provides a brief explanation of aerobic and anaerobic training, and why each is important. For those who are interested in doing more reading on it, I will suggest some excellent resources.

Aerobic versus Anaerobic

Let's start with some basic definitions:

- Aerobic energy system: An energy system that utilizes oxygen and stored fat to power physical activity. This system can support activity for prolonged periods, as stored fat and oxygen are available in almost endless supply. Even a highly trained triathlete with a body fat percentage in the single digits has more than enough stored fat for several Iron-distance races, back-to-back.

- Anaerobic energy system: An energy system that utilizes glycogen (stored sugar) to power physical activity. This system can support activity for relatively short periods of time, as the body stores sugar in relatively small quantities.

It is a common misunderstanding that lower levels of activity (at lower heart rates) are supported fully by the aerobic system. Likewise, many believe that as activity level (and heart rate) increases, we eventually reach a point (the anaerobic threshold), where the aerobic system shuts off and the anaerobic system takes over.

This is not what actually happens. In reality we are always fueled by both of these energy systems at the same time. It's only the ratio of the two systems that changes as the activity level changes. The intensity of our activity determines the ratio at which we are drawing from each system. At high levels of activity, we draw mostly from our anaerobic system; at low levels of activity we draw most from our aerobic system. But we are always drawing from both.

Heart rate is an excellent indicator of where we are in the spectrum of ratios of aerobic to anaerobic. At low heart rates, the mix is primarily aerobic. As our heart rate increases (because the level of effort increases), the mix becomes more and more anaerobic. At a certain point, what some refer to as the anaerobic threshold, the mix becomes more anaerobic than aerobic.

Most Iron-distance triathletes tend to train at a much higher heart rate than is optimal. The Iron-distance is an aerobic race, and the training therefore needs to be primarily aerobic. As you may note in the 30-week training programs, the maximum portion of anaerobic training in a given week is only about 10% of the total training, and usually it's much less than that. A full 90% or more of our Ironman training is going to be aerobic.

Below I will explain how to calculate your own heart rate training zones, and how to use them with the 30-week training programs in Chapter 7. While the proper zones vary from athlete to athlete, I will show you a reliable method for estimating your individual heart rate training zones. This will help to ensure highly efficient training.

Should I "Train How I Feel"?

As long as I can remember, I have heard endurance sports enthusiasts say that you should just "train how you feel." The belief behind this advice is that your body will naturally gravitate to the pace and effort level best for you.

Unfortunately, I find this isn't true. Most athletes who let their bodies determine their pace end up doing most of their training at less than fully effective heart rates. This results in "junk miles." They are not getting the maximum benefit out of their limited training time.

Even most who use a heart rate monitor tend to regard it merely as interesting information and not as a guide to the effort they should be exerting. Most athletes train at a pace that just "feels right." The problem is that, compared to heart rate, "feel" is not a reliable indicator. Feelings can be misleading, while the heart rate never lies.

It's important to train both the aerobic and anaerobic systems, although for Iron-distance training the aerobic system is by far the most important. In my experience, the best way to train them is to train them separately. Most training time (90% or more) needs to focus on aerobic system training, with less than 10% targeting the anaerobic system. We target each system by training within a precise range of heart rates. In between these fairly narrow ranges is a no-man's-land, too fast and too slow for optimum training of either system. We must be careful to avoid this in-between zone, as it is not effective for the Iron-distance and it can lead to performance stagnation. As we will see later in this Chapter, this no man's land of Iron-distance training is referred to as Zone 3 (Z3).

Ironically, this is where most athletes end up spending most of their training time. Why? For most athletes, aerobic system training seems too easy and comfortable. They doubt it is beneficial because it doesn't hurt enough. On the other hand, the high-intensity training that develops the anaerobic system is very uncomfortable; it takes great focus and discipline to maintain this level of effort for any period of time. Athletes training "by feel" tend to push beyond the aerobic training zone but not quite all the way up to the anaerobic training zone, because it's so unpleasant. They end up in this middle zone (Z3) because it feels like a good effort, but it's not too uncomfortable.

Effective heart rate training prevents us from training in the wrong zone, and it ensures that all of our training is beneficial and time efficient.

Should I Train at "My Pace"?

Some athletes believe they have what they refer to as "my pace." This is the time-measured pace at which they feel most comfortable, and which they try to maintain no matter what their heart rate is telling them. Just like training by feel, training by pace can also lead to junk miles and ineffective training.

I recommend giving up the concept of "my pace." It should be your goal to make a full range of paces "my pace." Pace is simply not a reliable indicator of how hard you are working. Many external factors, such as heat, hills, wind, altitude, insufficient sleep, etc., can affect the effort level required to maintain a certain pace. On a cool day, an 8-minutes-per-mile pace may be an aerobic effort; on a very hot day it may be an anaerobic effort. All of the above-mentioned factors could have this effect on heart rate.

What is the right indicator? Heart rate. Your heart rate doesn't lie. It will tell you how hard you are working. And what's more, it will automatically make all of the necessary adjustments for heat, wind, hills, altitude, a bad day—whatever. Heart rate, not pace, should be your primary indicator of training intensity.

Mileage Junkies

Another common training mistake is to schedule your training in miles and not in time. All of the 30-week IronFit training programs presented in this book are based on time, more specifically, time in the proper heart rate zone.

Many athletes get emotionally attached to their weekly mileage numbers. They are jokingly referred to as "mileage junkies." For them, achieving a weekly mileage goal becomes more important than the quality of the time spent training. No matter what, they are determined to achieve that magic number.

I have a friend who is an admitted mileage junkie. She has actually left her bed with a fever to complete her weekly mileage goal. She knows that the effort will probably hurt her long-term race goals more than help them, but she can't help herself.

I recommend forgetting about miles altogether. Run time, not miles. Going out for a 60-minute run in your aerobic heart rate zone is almost always better than going out for "8 miles at my pace."

As we've seen, the other great benefit of running time instead of miles is that it allows you to manage your training time more easily. A 60-minute run takes 60 minutes.

If you are like me, you will feel liberated when you give up mileage for "time in the zone." You will end up with higher-quality training, plus it's great fun when someone asks you how many miles you ran last week to answer "5 hours."

Calculating Your Heart Rate Zones

Now let's see how to calculate your personal heart rate zones, which will then be used in conjunction with the 30-week training programs presented in Chapter 7.

The most accurate way to determine your training heart rate zones is to have them formally tested. If you are interested in doing this, contact a local university with a sports medicine area to see if they offer this service to the public.

For many of us this is not possible or practical. Fortunately, you can reliably estimate your heart rate training zones using a lower-tech method. We begin by determining maximum heart rate, and then identify the various training ranges as percentages of the maximum.

The most generally accepted technique for estimating your maximum heart rate is the "220 Minus Your Age" method. Simply subtract your age from 220; the result is an estimate of your maximum heart rate.

Once we have this number, we can usually identify four distinct heart rate zones. The 30-week training programs incorporate these zones:

Zone 4: 90–95% of maximum heart rate (primarily anaerobic training)

Zone 3: 86–89% of maximum heart rate (middle zone)

Zone 2: 75–85% of maximum heart rate (higher-end aerobic training)

Zone 1: 65–74% of maximum heart rate (lower-end aerobic training)

Now let's take an example. Suppose you are a 35-year-old athlete. What are your training zones?

Your maximum heart rate is 220–35 years = 185 beats per minute (BPM). Using that number:

Z4: 90–95% of 185 BPM = 166 BPM to 175 BPM

Z3: 86–89% of 185 BPM = 159 to 165 BPM

Z2: 75–85% of 185 BPM = 139 to 158 BPM

Z1: 65–74% of 185 BPM = 120 to 138 BPM

After making your initial calculations based on the "220 Minus Your Age" rule, you may want to test them under real conditions and fine-tune them if necessary.

The best way to do this is to run a time trial of about 3 miles (Note: always do a 10–15 min. warm-up before and a 10–15 min. cool down after time trial tests.) Wear a heart rate monitor for a 3-mile time trial, or better yet a 5K race and observe your heart rate. If you put out a 100% effort at an even pace, your heart rate should climb above 90% of maximum (above the bottom of Z4) within the first mile, and you will reach your maximum heart rate in the final mile. If your results from the time trial differ from the estimates, adjust your heart rate zones according to the real-world result.

Because cycling stresses your body in different ways than running, I recommend that you subtract 5% when applying these heart rate zones to biking. In other words, when biking you obtain the equivalent training effect at a heart rate about 5% slower than when running. For example, let's now apply the 95% rule to the 35-year-old athlete we considered above to determine his or her proper heart rate zones for training on the bike:

RUNNING ZONES	BIKING ZONES
Z1 = 120–138 BPM	Z1 = 114–131 BPM
Z2 = 139–158 BPM	Z2 = 132–150 BPM
Z3 = 159–165 BPM	Z3 = 151–157 BPM
Z4 = 166–175 BPM	Z4 = 158–166 BPM

You may also want to test these estimated bike zones against a real-world result. To do so, perform a 15-minute time trial wearing a heart rate monitor. (Do this test in a flat, safe area with no traffic. Also, always do a 10–15 min. warm-up before and a 10–15 min. cool down after time trial tests.) If you give a 100% effort and cycle at an even pace, your heart rate should climb above 90% of maximum (above the bottom of Z4) within the first 5 minutes, and you will reach your maximum heart rate in the final 5 minutes. If your test results differ from the estimates, adjust your heart rate zones accordingly.

Additional information on estimating maximum heart rates is presented in Appendix D.

IRONFIT PROFILE

Steve Listzwan (written in 2004)

Steve Listzwan is a great example of someone who has become a rising star in the sport of triathlon while also excelling professionally. At thirty-two, Steve is a project manager at Merck, the world's largest pharmaceutical company. Steve's normal workday is 8 a.m. to 7 p.m., with frequent evening and weekend work and even some occasional international travel. With commuting time, Steve's workweek is at least 60 hours, and it can sometimes be 70 or more.

Steve had some background in cycling and rowing, but not until 1999 did he complete his first multisport race, a sprint-distance duathlon. Well, Steve got a taste of multisport racing and that's all it took. He had always been intrigued by the Hawaii Ironman, which he had seen many times on television. After his first sprint-distance triathlon, he immediately went out and signed up for the 2000 Ironman USA in Lake Placid.

Consistent with his usual no-nonsense approach to things, Steve read most of the training books out there, joined a Masters swim program (as a self-proclaimed Guppy), and signed up for online coaching (with me). Steve stuck with his training program, which ranged from 15 to 20 hours per week through most of the early months of 2000, and peaked at 20 hours per week for a couple of weeks during the key pre-race training period. Steve used other races through the first half of 2000 to help prepare him for his Iron-distance race in late July. These included a half-marathon in March; various sprint-distance duathlons in April and May; and a Half Iron-distance in early June, Eagleman, in Cambridge, Maryland.

On July 29, in his first Iron-distance—and only his second triathlon!—Steve raced to an incredible finish in 10 hours and 37 minutes. He was thrilled by his performance and deeply affected by the journey he had taken. Not surprisingly, Steve next set his long-term sights on making it to "The Show," the Hawaii Ironman World Championships.

Now let's look at Steve Listzwan's time-management successes. There are 168 hours in a week. Steve's minimum workweek is 60 and his weekly hours of sleep are about 51 (7 hours a day during the week and 8 hours a day on the weekends). Steve's maximum training week is 20 hours, leaving as little as 37 hours for meals, dressing, shopping, household chores, social time, etc. Not much, but I think you would agree that it is doable. Especially, when you are talking about living your dream.

Following are some of the time-saving techniques that Steve uses:

Lunchtime Training: Steve considers himself fortunate to have a fitness facility on-site, and he takes advantage of it. He averages three lunchtime workouts per week, and sometimes does as many as five; this is 3 to 5 quality hours added to his weekly training. Surely with the long hours he works, his boss should not have a problem with him taking a midday workout break; in fact, Steve comes back to work after these sessions recharged and more effective.

Train Early on Weekends: Instead of procrastinating and risking some surprise coming up during the day, Steve completes his weekend training early in the day, freeing up the remainder of the day for other activities.

Schedule Training Sessions in Day Planner: Steve actually writes his training sessions into his daily planner in advance, just like any other event or business meeting that is important to him. By doing this, he always allows sufficient time for his workouts.

Make Multiple Copies of Training Plan: Steve makes three copies of his training schedule, which he receives from his coach (me!) every 4 weeks. He posts one copy on his refrigerator and puts the others in his briefcase and at his desk. By doing this, Steve always knows what he needs to be scheduling around for the next several days, and is therefore always able to make plans that will fit his training schedule.

Set Up Clothes and Equipment the Evening Before: Steve doesn't usually train first thing in the morning; however, when he does, he lays out the clothes and equipment he will need. This allows him to be more efficient in the morning and not waste time looking for clothes and equipment.

Masters Swimming: Steve finds that his Masters program makes swim training very efficient. It has a specific time, so he can plan it right into his schedule. Another advantage is that he does not need to think up a workout or remember a workout from the training schedule he receives from his coach. All he has to do is show up. He finds that once he is there, the coach and the peer pressure from the other swimmers take over, and he is guaranteed an hour of quality swimming.

Family Meeting: Steve talked with his friends and family many months in advance of his first Ironman race to prepare them for the training hours to come and to ask for their support. It worked well: They all became very supportive of his goal and were well prepared when the long training days came.

"Work Family" Meeting: Steve found this relationship to be trickier. He has come to an understanding with his boss. Many of his coworkers, however, don't understand his commitment to triathlon, and some see it in a negative light, suspecting that his work must suffer. As a result Steve often prefers not to talk about triathlon with his colleagues.

Controlling Moods: Steve makes an effort to manage his moods. He sometimes feels a little worn down and grumpy after long training sessions and long workdays. Sometimes he doesn't even realize it. The family meeting helped a great deal in this regard. When people are told in advance what is to come, they are much more understanding. Steve finds that eating well and getting enough rest are helpful in avoiding bad moods.

Steve has gained from the Iron-distance experience in many ways. He has learned a new appreciation for time. Athletic training helps him to deal with stress and keep the daily ups and downs of life in perspective. Steve finds that he thinks more clearly when he is training, solving problems more easily and thinking more creatively. Overall, Steve believes that success in one area of life leads to success in others. Training for and racing the Iron-distance can build a pattern of success that expands into other areas of your life.

CHAPTER 7

30-Week IronFit Training Programs

"Now I only have two kinds of days . . .
good days and great days."

—*Lance Armstrong*

This chapter presents three 30-week training programs to prepare you for the Iron-distance. These detailed plans, together with the knowledge you will gain in this book, will arm you with everything you will need to accomplish your goal.

The programs are based on training time. The "Competitive Program" requires an average of about 12 hours per week of actual training, with a maximum week of 20 hours. The "Just Finish Program" averages only about 7 hours per week of training, with a peak week of 10 hours. For those who feel their possible time commitment will probably be somewhere between these two programs, there is the "Intermediate Program," which averages about 10.5 hours per week in training and peaks with 15 hours.

Although I will review and explain each program here, you will only be ready to select the plan best suited for you after you have familiarized yourself with all of the information in this book.

Each 30-week program has a similar format. All are constructed in three 10-week phases: the "Base Phase," the "Build Phase," and the "Peak Phase." Each program also includes seventeen swim workouts, with five or six designed specifically for each of the three phases.

Below I define the abbreviations used in the training programs and then explain some sample workouts.

Wk 1: Week 1

Z1, Z2, Z4: Heart rate zone 1, heart rate zone 2, heart rate zone 4 (I explain how to calculate your zones in Chapter 6).

0:30: 30 minutes

100+ RPM: High RPM Spin Session. Pedal bike at 100 or more pedal revolutions per minute.

Trans: Transition Workout, a combined bike/run session where we transition from cycling to running in 3 minutes or less (transition sessions are discussed in Chapter 3).

QC: Quick Change, the up-to-3-minute time period between the cycling and running portions of the Transition Workout.

Z1 to Z2: Train at a heart rate anywhere within zone 1 or zone 2. In these sessions, the athlete should decide the heart rate to train at within Z1 and Z2 based on feel. If the athlete feels rested and energized, he or she may want to select a heart rate in the Z2 range. If on the other hand, the athlete feels tired and low energy, he or she may want to select a heart rate in the Z1 range.

PU: Pick ups are short (30–60 seconds in length) increases in speed. The athlete will temporarily increase his/her speed to a level that would normally cause their heart rate to increase to Z4, had it been sustained for a longer period. Since the Pick up is for only a brief period (30–60 seconds in length), the athlete's heart rate does not rise above Z2.

Spin: Easy cycling in a low gear in order to recover from a strenuous effort.

Jog: Easy running at a slow pace in order to recover from a strenuous effort.

Sample Run or Bike Session: 0:30 Z2 (at 0:20, insert 5 min Z4): Begin this 30-minute session in your Z2 heart rate zone. At 20 minutes into the session, increase your heart rate to Z4 for 5 minutes by increasing your pace. Then return to Z2 for the remaining 5 minutes of the session.

Sample Bike Session: 0:45 Z2 (at 0:10, insert 5 x 1 min PU @ 1 min Spin): Begin this 45-minute bike session at a pace that will maintain a Z2 heart rate. At 10 minutes into the session, increase pace for 1 minute and then shift to an easier gear for an easy 1-minute Spin. Repeat this sequence five times, and then return to a Z2 heart rate for the remainder of the 45-minute ride.

Sample Run Session: 0:45 Z2 (at 0:10, insert 4 x 6 min Z4 @ 2 min Jog): Begin your 45-minute run at a pace that will maintain a Z2 heart rate. At 10 minutes into run, increase your pace enough to produce a Z4 heart rate for a period of 6 minutes. After the 6 minutes, slow down to an easy jog for 2 minutes. Repeat this sequence four times and then return to a Z2 heart rate for the remainder of the run.

Bike Safety Check: This refers to the pre-race bike safety check presented in Chapter 13. While the following programs call for a bike safety check and a Z1 bike ride on the day before all races, it is recommended the athlete perform the bike safety check prior to every bike training session and race.

Following are the three 30-week training programs and full explanations of each.

The Competitive Program

This is our highest-volume program, with an average of about 12 hours per week and a peak week of 20 hours. The Competitive Program starts with 6 hours of training in the first week and builds to a peak of 20 hours in Week 27. Each week is built according to the training principles discussed in this book and presented in an efficient and understandable format.

The Competitive Program tends to be the most popular of the three, because after learning the time-management secrets in this book, even the busiest people can learn to squeeze out an average of 12 hours of weekly training. I can think of doctors, construction workers, lawyers, firemen, investment bankers, and nurses who have all followed this program. All achieved their Iron-distance goal as a result.

This is much more than a program simply to finish the race within regulation time. I have worked with many athletes who far exceeded their own expectations—first-timers who finished 2 hours faster than projected, repeat Ironmen who took more than an hour off their previous best, and experienced Ironmen who even won their age group in the World Championships—all with training plans very similar to the Competitive Program presented here.

If after reading this book you decide that the Competitive Program is for you, you can select your Iron-distance race and you will know exactly how to train every single day for the 30 weeks (seven months) leading up to it. The guesswork is virtually eliminated.

As an example of how to apply the plan, let's select Ironman USA in Lake Placid, New York, as our race. Ironman Lake Placid is usually held on the fourth weekend in July. By counting back 30 weeks, we see that we would begin our training in the first week of January. What a great way to start the year—to begin an IronFit journey.

The Competitive Program includes two training races as part of our preparation: an Olympic-distance triathlon in Week 18 and a Half Iron-distance triathlon in Week 22. We will discuss the use of training races in Chapter 10. Using the Lake Placid example, this would mean an Olympic-distance race during the first week of May and a Half Iron-distance race during the first week of June. All we need to do is to select two appropriate races to fit this (we will discuss how to do this in Chapter 10), and we are all set to go to work on our 30-week training program.

The following is a summary of each of the three 10-week phases for the Competitive Program (i.e., the Base Phase, the Build Phase, and the Peak Phase) and the actual training programs corresponding to each.

● Base Phase (Weeks 1–10) for the Competitive Program

The primary goals of this phase are to (1) acclimate the athlete to the type of training that will follow, (2) establish an aerobic base, and (3) develop technique.

As discussed in Chapter 5, it is important that we allow our bodies to adapt gradually to our training volume. Jumping into training too quickly is not recommended, as it can result in injury or an early setback. Our first week of the Competitive Program begins with only 2 hours in each of the three sports. This includes a total of eight training sessions: two swims, three bike sessions, and three runs.

The Base Phase is fully aerobic: All training takes place in heart rate zone 1 or 2. Thus, all training during these 10 weeks should be at a comfortable level of effort. As we have already discussed in Chapter 6, building our aerobic base is the foundation of Iron-distance training.

Because we are training at a comfortable pace, this is an excellent time to focus on efficient technique. Instead of worrying about pushing ourselves, we want to be thinking about being as efficient as possible in our form. In particular, the Z1 (100+ RPM) cycling sessions (discussed in Chapter 3) and the Drill Sets in our swimming sessions are specific technique workouts. Proper technique will be discussed in detail in Chapter 11.

During the Base Phase of the Competitive Program, we will also have one Transition Session each week, in which a bike ride is followed by a quick change to running, both to practice transition skills (discussed in Chapter

12) and to prepare ourselves to run well immediately after cycling. The run portion of this workout begins at only 15 minutes but gradually increases.

Our Long Bike session will begin at only 1 hour in Week 1 and then build to 2.75 hours in Week 10. Our Long Run begins at 45 minutes in Week 1 and builds to 1.25 hours in Week 10.

The total weekly training durations generally increase by 1 hour each week through this phase, with a pause and a 1-hour decrease every fourth week to allow sufficient recovery and adaptation before continuing to build. The Base Phase begins with 6 hours of total training in Week 1 and concludes with 11 hours in Week 10.

To sum up, the Base Phase:

- Begins with 6 hours per week and concludes with 11 hours per week;

- Averages 8.5 hours per week.

The following chart details the Base Phase of the Competitive Program.

NOTE: The 17 swim workouts referred to in the following charts can be found later in this chapter.

THE COMPETITIVE PROGRAM

BASE TRAINING PHASE: WEEKS 1–10

WK 1	SW	BIKE	RUN
M		REST DAY	REST DAY
T	#1	Off	0:30 Z2
W		Trans: 0:30 Z2 (QC)	0:15 Z2
R	#2	0:30 Z1 (100+ RPM)	Off
F		Off	0:30 Z2
S		1:00 Z2	Off
S		Off	0:45 Z1 to Z2
Total Hrs:			
6:00	2:00	2:00	2:00

WK 2	SW	BIKE	RUN
M		REST DAY	REST DAY
T	#3	Off	0:30 Z2
W		Trans: 0:30 Z2 (QC)	0:15 Z2
R	#4	0:30 Z1 (100+ RPM)	Off
F		Off	0:45 Z2
S		1:30 Z2	Off
S		Off	1:00 Z1 to Z2
Total Hrs:			
7:00	2:00	2:30	2:30

WK 3	SW	BIKE	RUN
M		REST DAY	REST DAY
T	#5	Off	0:45 Z2
W		Trans: 0:30 Z2 (QC)	0:15 Z2
R	#1	0:45 Z1 (100+ RPM)	Off
F		Off	1:00 Z2
S		1:45 Z2	Off
S		Off	1:00 Z1 to Z2
Total Hrs:			
8:00	2:00	3:00	3:00

WK 4	SW	BIKE	RUN
M		REST DAY	REST DAY
T	#2	Off	0:30 Z2
W		Trans: 0:30 Z2 (QC)	0:15 Z2
R	#3	0:30 Z1 (100+ RPM)	Off
F		Off	0:45 Z2
S		1:30 Z2	Off
S		Off	1:00 Z1 to Z2
Total Hrs:			
7:00	2:00	2:30	2:30

WK 5	SW	BIKE	RUN
M		REST DAY	REST DAY
T	#4	Off	0:45 Z2
W		Trans: 0:30 Z2 (QC)	0:15 Z2
R	#5	0:45 Z1 (100+ RPM)	Off
F		Off	1:00 Z2
S		1:45 Z2	Off
S		Off	1:00 Z1 to Z2
Total Hrs:			
8:00	2:00	3:00	3:00

WK 6	SW	BIKE	RUN
M		REST DAY	REST DAY
T	#1	Off	1:00 Z2
W		Trans: 0:45 Z2 (QC)	0:15 Z2
R	#2	1:00 Z1 (100+ RPM)	Off
F		Off	1:00 Z2
S		2:00 Z2	Off
S		Off	1:00 Z1 to Z2
Total Hrs:			
9:00	2 :00	3:45	3:15

WK 7	SW	BIKE	RUN
M		REST DAY	REST DAY
T	#3	Off	1:00 Z2
W		Trans: 0:45 Z2 (QC)	0:15 Z2
R	#4	1:00 Z1 (100+ RPM)	Off
F		Off	1:15 Z2
S		2:30 Z2	Off
S		Off	1:15 Z1 to Z2
Total Hrs:			
10:00	2:00	4:15	3:45

WK 8	SW	BIKE	RUN
M		REST DAY	REST DAY
T	#5	Off	1:00 Z2
W		Trans: 0:45 Z2 (QC)	0:15 Z2
R	#1	1:00 Z1 (100+ RPM)	Off
F		Off	1:00 Z2
S		2:00 Z2	Off
S		Off	1:00 Z1 to Z2
Total Hrs:			
9:00	2:00	3:45	3:15

WK 9	SW	BIKE	RUN
M		REST DAY	REST DAY
T	#2	Off	1:00 Z2
W		Trans: 0:45 Z2 (QC)	0:15 Z2
R	#3	1:00 Z1 (100+ RPM)	Off
F		Off	1:00 Z2
S		2:45 Z2	Off
S		Off	1:15 Z1 to Z2
Total Hrs:			
10:00	2:00	4:30	3:30

WK 10	SW	BIKE	RUN
M		REST DAY	REST DAY
T	#4	Off	1:00 Z2
W		Trans: 0:45 Z2 (QC)	0:30 Z2
R	#5	1:15 Z1 (100+ RPM)	Off
F		Off	1:00 Z2
S		3:00 Z2	Off
S		Off	1:30 Z1 to Z2
Total Hrs:			
11:00	2:00	5:00	4:00

- **Build Phase (Weeks 11–20) for the Competitive Program**

The priorities in this phase are to build power and speed as we continue to gradually increase durations. At the conclusion of these 10 weeks, we will be prepared to take on the final peak preparation for our Iron-distance triathlon.

This phase begins with 12 hours in Week 11, and then builds to 16 hours in Week 20. While total durations only increase by 4 hours over this 10-week period, the training becomes gradually more intensive and challenging.

A third swim session is added each week and the sessions increase from about 2,500 yards/meters to about 3,000 yards/meters.

We gradually begin to include High Intensity Z4 sessions (discussed in Chapter 6) in both the run and the bike. In Week 12 these Z4 portions total only 15 minutes, or about 3% of our total cycling and running. This gradually increases each week, so that by Week 20 the Z4 portions total 60 minutes, or about 8% of our total cycling and running.

We add a second Transition Session each week to further develop our transition skills and our ability to run well after cycling.

Our Long Bike session increases to 4 hours, while our Long Run increases to 2 hours.

In Week 18 we have our first practice race. It is suggested that this be an Olympic-distance triathlon (1.5K swim, 40K bike, and 10K run), however, if a race of this distance is not available, you should find a race as close in distance as possible. Chapter 10 has tips on how to locate the right race for you.

Following this race, we have a week of pure aerobic training (Z1 and Z2) to recover and prepare for the work ahead.

To sum up, the Build Phase:

- Begins with 12 hours of training per week and concludes with 16 hours per week;

- Averages about 13 hours per week.

The following chart details the Build Phase of the Competitive Program.

THE COMPETITIVE PROGRAM

BUILD PHASE: WEEKS 11–20

WK 11	SW	BIKE	RUN
M		REST DAY	REST DAY
T	#6	Off	1:00 Z2 (at 0:10, insert 5 x 1 min PU @ 1 min Jog)
W		Trans: 0:45 Z2 (QC)	0:30 Z2
R	#7	1:15 Z2 (at 0:15, insert 5 x 1 min easy PU @ 1 min Spin)	Off
F	#8	Off	1:00 Z2 (at 0:45, insert 5 x 1 min PU @ 1 min Jog)
S		Trans: 2:30 Z2 (QC)	0:15 Z2
S		0:30 Z1 (100+ RPM)	1:15 Z1 to Z2
Total Hrs:			
12:00	3:00	5:00	4:00

WK 12	SW	BIKE	RUN
M		REST DAY	REST DAY
T	#9	Off	0:45 Z2 (at 0:10, insert 5 min Z4)
W		Trans: 0:45 Z2 (QC)	0:15 Z2
R	#10	1:00 Z2 (at 0:15, insert 5 min Z4)	Off
F	#11	Off	1:00 Z2 (at 0:45, insert 5 min Z4)
S		Trans: 2:30 Z2 (QC)	0:15 Z2
S		0:30 Z1 (100+ RPM)	1:00 Z1 to Z2
Total Hrs:			
11:00	3:00	4:45	3:15

WK 13	SW	BIKE	RUN
M		REST DAY	REST DAY
T	#6	Off	0:45 Z2 (at 0:10, insert 3 x 3 min Z4 @ 1 min Jog)
W		Trans: 0:45 Z2 (QC)	0:15 Z2
R	#7	1:00 Z2 (at 0:15, insert 2 x 5 min Z4 @ 3 min Spin)	Off
F	#8	Off	1:00 Z2 (at 0:45, insert 5 min Z4)
S		Trans: 3:00 Z2 (at 2:50, insert 5 min Z4) (QC)	0:30 Z2
S		0:30 Z1 (100+ RPM)	1:15 Z1 to Z2
Total Hrs:			
12:00	3:00	5:15	3:45

WK 14	SW	BIKE	RUN
M		REST DAY	REST DAY
T	#9	Off	1:00 Z2 (at 10 min, insert 2 x 4.5 min Z4 @ 1.5 min Jog)
W		Trans: 0:45 Z2 (QC)	0:30 Z2
R	#10	1:00 Z2 (at 15 min, insert 3 x 5 min Z4 @ 3 min Spin)	Off
F	#11	Off	1:00 Z2 (at 0:45, insert 7.5 min Z4)
S		Trans: 3:30 Z2 (at 3:20, insert 5 min Z4) (QC)	0:30 Z2
S		0:30 Z1 (100+ RPM)	1:15 Z1 to Z2
Total Hrs:			
13:00	3:00	5:45	4:15

WK 15	SW	BIKE	RUN
M		REST DAY	REST DAY
T	#6	Off	1:00 Z2 (at 10 min, insert 2 x 6 min Z4 @ 2 min Jog)
W		Trans: 0:45 Z2 (QC)	0:30 Z2
R	#7	1:00 Z2 (at 15 min, insert 4 x 5 min Z4 @ 3 min Spin)	Off
F	#8	Off	1:00 Z2 (at 45 min, insert 7.5 min Z4)
S		Trans: 4:00 Z2 (at 3:50, insert 5 min Z4) (QC)	0:30 Z2
S		0:45 Z1 (100+ RPM)	1:30 Z1 to Z2
Total Hrs:			
14:00	3:00	6:30	4:30

WK 16	SW	BIKE	RUN
M		REST DAY	REST DAY
T	#9	Off	1:00 Z2 (at 0:10, insert 5 x 3 min Z4 @ 1 min Jog)
W		Trans: 0:45 Z2 (QC)	0:30 Z2
R	#1	1:00 Z2 (at 0:15, insert 5 x 5 min Z4 @ 3 min Spin)	Off
F	#11	Off	1:00 Z2 (at 0:45, insert 10 min Z4)
S		Trans: 3:00 Z2 (at 2:50, insert 5 min Z4) (QC)	0:30 Z2
S		0:45 Z1 (100+ RPM)	1:30 Z1 to Z2
Total Hrs:			
13:00	3:00	5:30	4:30

WK 17	SW	BIKE	RUN
M		REST DAY	REST DAY
T	#6	Off	1:00 Z2 (at 0:10, insert 3 x 6 min Z4 @ 2 min Jog)
W		Trans: 0:45 Z2 (QC)	0:30 Z2
R	#7	1:15 Z2 (at 0:10, insert 6 x 5 min Z4 @ 3 min Spin)	Off
F	#8	Off	1:15 Z2 (at 1:00, insert 10 min Z4)
S		Trans: 3:30 Z2 (QC)	0:30 Z2
S		1:00 Z1 (100+ RPM)	1:15 Z1 to Z2
Total Hrs:			
14:00	3:00	6:30	4:30

WK 18	SW	BIKE	RUN
M		REST DAY	REST DAY
T	#9	Off	1:00 Z2 (at 0:10, insert 5 x 1 min easy PU @ 1 min Jog)
W		Trans: 0:45 Z2 (QC)	0:30 Z2
R	0:30 easy	1:00 Z1 (at 0:15, insert 5 x 1 min easy PU @ 1 min Spin)	Off
F		Off	0:40 Z1 (at 0:10, insert 5 x 1 min easy PU @ 1 min Jog)
S		0:15 Z1 – easy Bike Safety Check	0:20 Z1 – easy
S	Race	Race (Olympic distance) Optional: 2:00 hr Z1 – easy (in p.m.)	Race (Olympic distance)
Total Hrs:			
8:30 (+ Race)	2:00	4:00 (+ Race)	2:30 (+ Race)

WK 19	SW	BIKE	RUN
M		REST DAY	REST DAY
T	#10	Off	1:00 Z1 to Z2
W		Trans: 0:45 Z2 (QC)	0:30 Z2
R	#11	1:15 Z2	Off
F	#6	Off	1:15 Z2
S		Trans: 4:00 Z2 (QC)	0:45 Z2
S		1:00 Z1 (100+ RPM)	1:30 Z1 to Z2
Total Hrs:			
15:00	3:00	7:00	5:00

WK 20	SW	BIKE	RUN
M		REST DAY	REST DAY
T	#12	Off	1:00 Z2 (at 0:10, insert 4 x 4.5 min Z4 @ 1.5 min Jog)
W		Trans: 0:45 Z2 (QC)	0:30 Z2
R	#13	1:30 Z2 (at 0:15, insert 8 x 4 min Z4 @ 2 min Spin)	Off
F	#14	Off	1:15 Z2 (at 1:00, insert 10 min Z4)
S		Trans: 4:00 Z2 (QC)	0:45 Z2
S		1:15 Z1 (100+ RPM)	2:00 Z1 to Z2
Total Hrs:			
16:00	3:00	7:30	5:30

- **Peak Phase (Weeks 21–30) for the Competitive Program**

This phase begins with a Half Iron-distance triathlon (1.2-mile swim, 56-mile bike, and 13.1-mile run) as our final practice race. Then we go into the key 5-week intensive training volume buildup before the final 3-week pre-race taper—and then of course our Iron-distance race itself.

Weekly training durations start at 16 hours in Week 16 and build to a peak of 20 hours in Week 27. They then drop to 14.5 hours in Week 28, 11 hours in Week 29, and only 5 hours in the final week, not including the race.

The Half Iron-distance race is ideally placed 8 weeks before our Iron-distance triathlon. This serves as a final dress rehearsal before we go into the 5-week build/3-week taper mentioned above. This is a great opportunity to check our progress and learn what areas require extra focus over the final training period. Following the race we again have a week of pure aerobic training (Z1 and Z2) to recover and prepare for the work ahead.

Swim sessions generally increase from about 3,000 yards/meters to about 3,500 yards/meters. Our Long Bike session builds to a peak of 6 hours, while our Long Run session increases to a high of 3 hours. Our Z1 (100+ RPM) cycling technique sessions increase to 1.5 hours.

The High Intensity Z4 portion of our cycling and running starts in Week 21 at 56 minutes, or about 7% of our volume. In Week 27 we reach our greatest amount of Z4 work: 87 minutes, or about 9% of our total volume.

To sum up, the Peak Phase:

- Begins with 16 hours per week and peaks at 20 hours per week;

- Average: 15 hours per week.

The following chart details the Peak Phase of the Competitive Program:

THE COMPETITIVE PROGRAM

PEAK PHASE: WEEKS 21–30

WK 21	SW	BIKE	RUN
M		REST DAY	REST DAY
T	#15	Off	1:15 Z2 (at 0:10, insert 3 x 6 min Z4 @ 2 min Jog)
W		Trans: 0:45 Z2 (QC)	0:30 Z2

WK 21	SW	BIKE	RUN
R	#16	1:30 Z2 (at 0:15, insert 4 x 7 min Z4 @ 4 min Spin)	Off
F	#17	Off	1:15 Z2 (at 1:00, insert 10 min Z4)
S		Trans: 4:00 Z2 (QC)	0:45 Z2
S		1:15 Z1 (100+ RPM)	1:45 Z1 to Z2
Total Hrs:			
16:00	3:00	7:30	5:30

WK 22	SW	BIKE	RUN
M		REST DAY	REST DAY
T	#12	Off	1:00 Z2 (at 0:10, insert 5 x 1 min PU @ 1 min Jog)
W		Trans: 0:45 Z2 (QC)	0:30 Z2
R	0:30 easy	1:00 Z1 (at 0:15, insert 5 x 1 min PU @ 1 min Spin)	Off
F		Off	0:40 Z1 (at 0:10, insert 5 x 1 min PU @ 1 min Jog)
S		0:15 Z1 – easy Bike Safety Check	0:20 Z1 – easy
S	Race	Race (Half Iron-distance)	Race (Half Iron-distance)
Total Hrs:			
6:30 (+ Race)	2:00	2:00 (+ Race)	2:30 (+ Race)

WK 23	SW	BIKE	RUN
M		REST DAY	REST DAY
T	#13	Off	1:15 Z1 to Z2
W		Trans: 0:45 Z2 (QC)	0:30 Z2
R	#14	1:30 Z2	Off
F	#15	Off	1:30 Z2
S		Trans: 5:00 Z2 (QC)	0:45 Z2
S		0:45 Z1 (100+ RPM)	2:00 Z1 to Z2
Total Hrs.			
17:00	3:00	8:00	6:00

WK 24	SW	BIKE	RUN
M		REST DAY	REST DAY
T	#16	Off	1:15 Z2 (at 0:10, insert 3 x 6 min Z4 @ 2 min Jog)
W		Trans: 1:00 Z2 (QC)	0:30 Z2
R	#17	1:30 Z2 (at 1:10, insert 15 min Z4)	Off
F	#12	Off	1:30 Z2 (at 1:10, insert 10 min Z4)
S		Trans: 5:00 Z2 (at 4:45, insert 7.5 min Z4) (QC)	1:00 Z2
S		1:00 Z1 (100+ RPM)	2:15 Z1 to Z2
Total Hrs:			
18:00	3:00	8:30	6:30

WK 25	SW	BIKE	RUN
M		REST DAY	REST DAY
T	#13	Off	1:00 Z2 (at 0:10, insert 4 x 6 min Z4 @ 2 min Jog)
W		Trans: 1:00 Z2 (QC)	0:30 Z2
R	#14	1:30 Z2 (at 1:00, insert 20 min Z4)	Off
F	#15	Off	1:30 Z2 (at 1:10, insert 10 min Z4)
S		Trans: 5:30 Z2 (at 5:15, insert 10 min Z4) (QC)	1:00 Z2
S		1:30 Z1 (100+ RPM)	2:30 Z1 to Z2
Total Hrs:			
19:00	3:00	9:30	6:30

WK 26	SW	BIKE	RUN
M		REST DAY	REST DAY
T	#16	Off	1:00 Z2 (at 0:10, insert 5 x 6 min Z4 @ 2 min Jog)
W		Trans: 1:00 Z2 (QC)	0:30 Z2
R	#17	1:30 Z2 (at 0:55, insert 25 min Z4)	Off
F	#12	Off	1:30 Z2 (at 1:10, insert 12 min Z4)
S		Trans: 5:30 Z2 (at 5:10, insert 12 min Z4) (QC)	1:00 Z2
S		1:15 Z1 (100+ rpm)	2:45 Z1 to Z2
Total Hrs:			
19:30	3:00	9:45	6:45

WK 27	SW	BIKE	RUN
M		REST DAY	REST DAY
T	#13	Off	1:00 Z2 (at 0:10, insert 5 x 6 min Z4 @ 2 min Jog)
W		Trans: 1:00 Z2 (QC)	0:30 Z2
R	#14	1:30 Z2 (at 0:50, insert 30 min Z4)	Off
F	#15	Off	1:30 Z2 (at 1:10, insert 12 min Z4)
S		Trans 6:00 Z2 (at 5:40, insert 15 min Z4) (QC)	1:00 Z2
S		1:30 Z1 (100+ RPM)	3:00 Z1 to Z2
Total Hrs:			
20:00	3:00	10:00	7:00

WK 28	SW	BIKE	RUN
M		REST DAY	REST DAY
T	#16	Off	0:45 Z2 (at 0:10, insert 3 x 6 min Z4 @ 2 min Jog
W		Trans: 0:45 Z2 (QC)	0:30 Z2
R	#17	1:00 Z2 (at 0:40, insert 15 min Z4)	Off
F	#12	Off	1:00 Z2 (at 0:40, insert 10 min Z4)
S		Trans: 4:00 Z2 (at 3:45, insert 10 min Z4) (QC)	0:30 Z2
S		1:00 Z1 (100 + RPM)	2:00 Z1 to Z2
Total Hrs:			
14:30	3:00	6:45	4:45

WK 29	SW	BIKE	RUN
M		REST DAY	REST DAY
T	#13	Off	0:45 Z2 (at 0:10, insert 2 x 6 min Z4 @ 2 min Jog)
W		Trans: 0:45 Z2 (QC)	0:15 Z2
R	#14	1:00 Z2 (at 0:45, insert 10 min Z4)	Off
F	#15	Off	0:45 Z2 (at 0:30, insert 7.5 min Z4)
S		Trans: 2:00 Z2 (QC)	0:30 Z2
S		1:00 Z1 (100+ RPM)	1:00 Z1 to Z2
Total Hrs:			
11:00	3:00	4:45	3:15

WK 30	SW	BIKE	RUN
M		REST DAY	REST DAY
T	#16	Off	0:45 Z2 (at 0:10, insert 5 x 1 min PU @ 1 min Jog)
W		Trans: 0:45 Z2 (QC)	0:15 Z2
R	0:30 easy	1:00 Z1 (at 0:15, insert 5 x 1 min PU @ 1 min Spin)	Off
F		Off	0:40 Z1 (at 0:10, insert 5 x 1 min PU @ 1 min Jog)
S		0:15 Z1 – easy Bike Safety Check	0:20 Z1 – easy (in a.m.)
S	Race	Race – Iron-distance	Race – Iron-distance
Total Hrs:			
5:00 (+ **Race**)	1:00	2:00 (+ Race)	2:00 (+ Race)

- **Swimming Sessions for the Competitive Program**

Below are the seventeen swim sessions referred to by number in the swim (SW) column of the training schedules for each of the three phases of the Competitive Program. The following is an explanation of the abbreviations and terms used:

wu: Warm Up

cd: Cool Down

DR: Swim Drills

Pull: Done with pull buoy (i.e., no kicking).

Pool size: Either yards or meters is fine.

@20sec: Take 20 seconds of rest at the wall after each effort in the set.

Perceived Effort: Warm Up, Cool Down, and Drills should be performed at 65% to 70% perceived effort; Main Sets at 80% to 85% perceived effort.

Base Phase (Weeks 1–10) Swim Sessions (about 2,500 meters/yards)

1. 300wu, 8x50 DR, 12 x 100 @20sec, 8x50 DR, 200 cd

2. 300wu, 8x50 DR, 3 x 125 @20sec, 2 x 175 @30sec, 3 x 125 @20sec, 8x50 DR, 200 cd

3. 300wu, 8x50 DR, 16 x 25 @10sec, 1 x 400 @60sec, 16 x 25 @10 sec, 8x50 DR, 200 cd

4. 300wu, 8x50 DR, 1 x 300 @40sec, 3 x 200 @30sec, 1 x 300 @30sec, 8x50 DR, 200 cd

5. 2,500 straight swim at comfortable pace (75–80% perceived effort)

Build Phase (Weeks 11–20) Swim Sessions (about 3,000 meters/yards)

6. 500wu, 8x50 DR, 4 x 200 @20sec, 6 x 100 @15sec, 8x50 DR, 300 cd

7. 500wu, 8x50 DR, 16 x 25 @10sec, 600 Pull, 16 x 25 @10 sec, 8x50 DR, 300 cd

8. 500wu, 8x50 DR, 10 x 50 @15sec, 4 x 100 @20sec, 10 x 50 @15sec, 8x50 DR, 300 cd

9. 500wu, 8x50 DR, 200-300-400-500 @ 45sec, 8x50 DR, 300 cd

10. 500wu, 8x50 DR, 7 x 125 @20sec, 7 x 75 @15sec, 8x50 DR, 300 cd

11. 3,000 straight swim at comfortable pace (75–80% perceived effort)

Peak Phase (Weeks 21–30) Swim Sessions (about 3,500 meters/yards)

12. 500 wu, 8x50 DR, 12 x 75 @20sec, 12 x 50 @15sec, 12 x 25 @10sec, 8x50 DR, 300 cd

13. 500 wu, 8x50 DR, 5 x 400 @45sec, 8x50 DR, 300 cd

14. 500 wu, 8x50 DR, 6 x (50+100+150) @20sec, 8x50 DR, 300 cd

15. 500 wu, 8x50 DR, 5 x 200 @30sec, 5 x 100 @20sec, 5 x 50 @10sec, 6 x 25 @5sec, 8x50 DR, 300 cd

16. 500 wu, 8x50 DR, 3 x 150 @20sec, 4 x 250 @30sec, 3 x 150 @20sec, 8x50 DR, 300 cd

17. 3,500 straight swim at comfortable pace (75–80% perceived effort)

The "Just Finish" Program

The "Just Finish" Program is for the super-busy athlete. Even with all the time-management techniques in this book, this aspiring Iron-distance triathlete can only squeeze out an average of about 7 hours per week over the 30-week training period, and then a few peak weeks of 10 hours per week during the final build-up. This athlete is not looking to break the course record. His or her goal is to complete an Iron-distance race within the regulation time, and to do it in good health and good spirits.

Like the Competitive Program, the Just Finish Program also incorporates two strategically placed practice races, and it packs all of the necessary training elements into the minimum amount of training time.

The following is a summary of each of the three 10-week phases for the Just Finish Program (the Base Phase, the Build Phase, and the Peak Phase) and the actual training programs, corresponding to each.

• Base Phase (Weeks 1–10) for the Just Finish Program

The Base Phase begins with only 3 hours of training in Week 1. Just 1 hour in each sport spread over eight workout sessions: three bikes, three runs, and two swims. From there, each week builds by between 30 and 45 minutes. By Week 10 we total close to 7 hours of total training, with the same number of workouts.

As in the Competitive Program, our priorities in the Base Phase are to (1) acclimate the athlete to the type of training we will be doing, (2) establish an aerobic base, and (3) build technique.

Also like the Competitive Program, the Base Phase in this program is fully aerobic (discussed in Chapter 6) and should feel very comfortable. This comfortable pace affords an excellent opportunity to work on improving technique (discussed in Chapter 11).

Our Long Bike starts in Week 1 at 30 minutes and builds to 2 hours in Week 10. Meanwhile, our Long Run starts at 30 minutes and increases to 1.5 hours in Week 10.

We will swim two sessions per week, each about 1,600 yards/meters in distance; of this, 800 yards/meters will focus on technique drills.

At 6 weeks into the Base Phase we will introduce one Transition Session per week (discussed in Chapter 3) for the purpose of practicing our transition skills (discussed in Chapter 12) and to prepare to run well immediately after cycling.

To sum up, the Base Phase:

- Begins with 3 hours per week and concludes with close to 7 hours per week;

- Averages about 5 hours per week.

The following chart details the Base Phase of the Just Finish Program.

THE JUST FINISH PROGRAM

BASE PHASE: WEEKS 1–10

WK 1	SW	BIKE	RUN
M		REST DAY	REST DAY
T	#18	Off	0:15 Z2
W		0:15 Z2	Off
R		0:15 Z2	Off
F	#19	Off	0:15 Z2
S		0:30 Z2	Off
S		Off	0:30 Z1 to Z2
Total Hrs:			
3:00	1:00	1:00	1:00

WK 2	SW	BIKE	RUN
M		REST DAY	REST DAY
T	#20	Off	0:30 Z2
W		0:30 Z2	Off
R		0:15 Z2	Off
F	#21	Off	0:15 Z2
S		0:30 Z2	Off
S		Off	0:30 Z1 to Z2
Total Hrs:			
3:30	1:00	1:15	1:15

WK 3	SW	BIKE	RUN
M		REST DAY	REST DAY
T	#22	Off	0:30 Z2
W		0:30 Z2	Off
R		0:30 Z2	Off
F	#18	Off	0:30 Z2
S		0:30 Z2	Off
S		Off	0:30 Z1 to Z2
Total Hrs:			
4:00	1:00	1:30	1:30

WK 4	SW	BIKE	RUN
M		REST DAY	REST DAY
T	#19	Off	0:30 Z2
W		0:30 Z2	Off
R		0:30 Z2	Off
F	#20	Off	0:15 Z2
S		0:30 Z2	Off
S		Off	0:30 Z1 to Z2
Total Hrs:			
3:45	1:00	1:30	1:15

WK 5	SW	BIKE	RUN
M		REST DAY	REST DAY
T	#21	Off	0:30 Z2
W		0:30 Z2	Off
R		0:30 Z2	Off
F	#22	Off	0:30 Z2
S		0:45 Z2	Off
S		Off	0:30 Z2
Total Hrs:			
4:15	1:00	1:45	1:30

WK 6	SW	BIKE	RUN
M		REST DAY	REST DAY
T	#18	Off	0:30 Z2
W		Trans: 0:30 Z2 (QC)	0:15 Z2
R		0:30 Z2	Off
F	#19	Off	Off
S		1:15 Z2	Off
S		Off	0:45 Z1 to Z2
Total Hrs:			
4:45	1:00	2:15	1:30

WK 7	SW	BIKE	RUN
M		REST DAY	REST DAY
T	#20	Off	0:30 Z2
W		Trans: 0:30 Z2 (QC)	0:15 Z2
R		0:45 Z2	Off
F	#21	Off	Off
S		1:30 Z2	Off
S		Off	1:00 Z1 to Z2
Total Hrs:			
5:30	1:00	2:45	1:45

WK 8	SW	BIKE	RUN
M		REST DAY	REST DAY
T	#22	Off	0:30 Z2
W		Trans: 0:30 Z2 (QC)	0:15 Z2
R		0:30 Z2	Off
F	#18	Off	Off
S		1:30 Z2	Off
S		Off	1:00 Z1 to Z2
Total Hrs:			
5:15	1:00	2:30	1:45

WK 9	SW	BIKE	RUN
M		REST DAY	REST DAY
T	#19	Off	0:30 Z2
W		Trans: 0:30 Z2 (QC)	0:15 Z2
R		0:45 Z2	Off
F	#20	Off	Off
S		1:45 Z2	Off
S		Off	1:15 Z1 to Z2
Total Hrs:			
6:00	1:00	3:00	2:00

WK 10	SW	BIKE	RUN
M		REST DAY	REST DAY
T	#21	Off	0:45 Z2
W		Trans: 0:30 Z2 (QC)	0:15 Z2
R		0:45 Z2	Off
F	#22	Off	Off
S		2:00 Z2	Off
S		Off	1:30 Z1 to Z2
Total Hrs:			
6:45	1:00	3:15	2:30

- **Build Phase (Weeks 11–20) for the Just Finish Program**

As with the Competitive Program, the Build Phase for the Just Finish Program focuses on building power and speed as we continue to gradually increase durations. At the conclusion of these 10 weeks, we will be prepared to take on the final peak preparation for our Iron-distance race.

This phase begins with about 7 hours of training in Week 11 and then builds to about 9 hours in Week 20. While total durations only increase by 2 hours over this 10-week period, the training becomes gradually more intensive and challenging.

The number of swim sessions per week remains at two; however, the length of the sessions increases from about 1,600 yards/meters to about 2,400 yards/meters.

Our Long Bike increases to 3 hours, while our Long Run builds to 2 hours.

We gradually introduce High Intensity Z4 sessions (discussed in Chapter 3 and 6) in both the run and the bike. In Week 12 these Z4 portions total only 10 minutes, or about 3% of our total cycling and running. This portion gradually increases each week, rising in Week 17 to 24 minutes, or about 6% of our total cycling and running.

In Week 18 we have our first practice race (discussed in Chapter 10). It is suggested that this be an Olympic-distance triathlon (1.5K swim, 40K bike, and 10K run). If a race of this distance is not available, you should find a race as close in distance as possible. Chapter 10 has tips on how to locate the right race for you.

Following our race, we have a week of pure aerobic training (Z1 and Z2) to recover and prepare for the work ahead.

To sum up, the Build Phase:

- Begins with about 7 hours per week and concludes with about 9 hours per week;

- Averages about 8 hours per week.

The following chart details the Build Phase of the Just Finish Program.

THE JUST FINISH PROGRAM

BUILD PHASE: WEEKS 11–20

WK 11	SW	BIKE	RUN
M		REST DAY	REST DAY
T	#23	Off	0:45 Z2 (at 0:10, insert 5 x 1 min PU @ 1 min Jog)
W		Trans: 0:30 Z2 (QC)	0:15 Z2
R		1:00 Z2 (at 0:45, insert 5 x 1 min PU @ 1 min Spin)	Off

WK 11	SW	BIKE	RUN
F	#24	Off	Off
S		2:00 Z2	Off
S		Off	1:15 Z1 to Z2
Total Hrs:			
7:15	1:30	3:30	2:15

WK 12	SW	BIKE	RUN
M		REST DAY	REST DAY
T	#25	Off	0:45 Z2 (at 0:10, insert 5 min Z4)
W		Trans: 0:30 Z2 (QC)	0:15 Z2
R		1:00 Z2 (at 0:45, insert 5 min Z4)	Off
F	#26	Off	Off
S		2:00 Z2	Off
S		Off	1:00 Z1 to Z2
Total Hrs:			
7:00	1:30	3:30	2:00

WK 13	SW	BIKE	RUN
M		REST DAY	REST DAY
T	#27	Off	0:45 Z2 (at 0:30, insert 5 min Z4)
W		Trans: 0:30 Z2 (QC)	0:15 Z2
R		1:00 Z2 (at 0:45, insert 5 min Z4)	Off
F	#23	Off	Off
S		2:00 Z2	Off
S		Off	1:15 Z1 to Z2
Total Hrs:			
7:15	1:30	3:30	2:15

WK 14	SW	BIKE	RUN
M		REST DAY	REST DAY
T	#24	Off	0:45 Z2 (at 0:30, insert 7.5 min Z4)
W		Trans: 0:30 Z2 (QC)	0:15 Z2
R		1:00 Z2 (at 0:45, insert 7.5 min Z4)	Off
F	#25	Off	Off
S		2:15 Z2	Off
S		Off	1:30 Z1 to Z2
Total Hrs:			
7:45	1:30	3:45	2:30

WK 15	SW	BIKE	RUN
M		REST DAY	REST DAY
T	#26	Off	0:45 Z2 (at 0:10, insert 7.5 min Z4)
W		Trans: 0:30 Z2 (QC)	0:15 Z2
R		1:00 Z2 (at 0:45, insert 7.5 min Z4)	Off
F	#27	Off	Off
S		2:30 Z2	Off
S		Off	1:30 Z1 to Z2
Total Hrs:			
8:00	1:30	4:00	2:30

WK 16	SW	BIKE	RUN
M		REST DAY	REST DAY
T	#23	Off	0:45 Z2 (at 0:30, insert 10 min Z4)
W		Trans: 0:30 Z2 (QC)	0:15 Z2
R		1:00 Z2 (at 0:45, insert 10 min Z4)	Off
F	#24	Off	Off

WK 16	SW	BIKE	RUN
S		2:30 Z2	Off
S		Off	1:15 Z1 to Z2
Total Hrs:			
7:45	1:30	4:00	2:15

WK 17	SW	BIKE	RUN
M		REST DAY	REST DAY
T	#25	Off	1:00 Z2 (at 0:40, insert 12 min Z4)
W		Trans: 0:30 Z2 (QC)	0:15 Z2
R		1:00 Z2 (at 0:40, insert 12 min Z4)	Off
F	#26	Off	Off
S		2:30 Z2	Off
S		Off	1:30 Z1 to Z2
Total Hrs:			
8:15	1:30	4:00	2:45

WK 18	SW	BIKE	RUN
M		REST DAY	REST DAY
T	#27	Off	1:00 Z2 (at 0:45, insert 5 x 1 min PU @ 1 min Jog
W		Trans: 0:30 Z2 (QC)	0:15 Z2
R	0:30 easy	1:00 Z1 (at 0:45, insert 5 x 1 min PU @ 1 min Spin)	Off
F		Off	Off
S		0:15 Z1 – easy Bike Safety Check	0:15 Z1 – easy PU
S	Race	Race (Olympic distance)	Race (Olympic distance)
Total Hrs:			
4:45 (+Race)	1:30+R	1:45 (+Race)	1:30 (+Race)

WK 19	SW	BIKE	RUN
M		REST DAY	REST DAY
T	#23	Off	1:00 Z1 to Z2
W		Trans: 0:30 Z2 (QC)	0:15 Z2
R		1:00 Z2	Off
F	#24	Off	Off
S		3:00 Z2	Off
S		Off	2:00 Z1 to Z2
Total Hrs:			
9:15	1:30	4:30	3:15

WK 20	SW	BIKE	RUN
M		REST DAY	REST DAY
T	#25	Off	1:00 Z2 (at 0:40, insert 15 min Z4)
W		Trans: 0:45 Z2 (QC)	0:15 Z2
R		1:00 Z2 (at 0:40, insert 15 min Z4)	Off
F	#26	Off	Off
S		3:00 Z2	Off
S		Off	1:45 Z1 to Z2
Total Hrs:			
9:15	1:30	4:45	3:00

• Peak Phase (Weeks 21–30) of the Just Finish Program

This phase begins with a Half Iron-distance triathlon (1.2-mile swim, 56-mile bike, and 13.1-mile run), our final practice race. We then enter the key 6-week intensive training volume buildup, before the final 2-week pre-race taper, and of course, the Iron-distance race itself.

Weekly training durations start at a peak of 10 hours in Week 21 and remain there through Week 28. We then drop to 7.5 hours in Week 29 and only 4 hours in the final week, not including our race.

As in the Competitive Program, the Half Iron-distance race is ideally placed 8 weeks before our Iron-distance. This serves as sort of a final dress rehearsal before we go into the final 6-week build/2-week taper mentioned above. This is a great opportunity to check our progress and learn what areas require extra focus over the final training period.

Again, following our race, we have a week of pure aerobic training (Z1 and Z2) to recover and prepare for the work ahead.

We continue with two swim sessions per week; most remain at about 2,400 yards/meters, although three longer sessions are at 3,500 yards/meters.

Our Long Bike session builds to a maximum of 5 hours. Our Long Run increases to a peak of 3 hours.

The High Intensity Z4 portion of our cycling and running starts in Week 21 at 20 minutes, or about 4% of our volume. In Week 27 we reach our greatest amount of Z4 work: 45 minutes, or about 8% of our total volume.

To sum up, the Peak Phase:

- Begins with 10 hours per week and remains at that peak for 8 weeks;

- Averages about 9 hours per week.

The following chart details the Peak Phase of the Just Finish Program.

THE JUST FINISH PROGRAM

PEAK PHASE: WEEKS 21–30

WK 21	SW	BIKE	RUN
M		REST DAY	REST DAY
T	#28	Off	1:00 Z2 (at 0:45, insert 10 min Z4)
W		Trans: 0:30 Z2 (QC)	0:15 Z2
R		1:00 Z2 (at 0:45, insert 10 min Z4)	Off
F	#29	Off	Off

WK 21	SW	BIKE	RUN
S		3:45 Z2	Off
S		Off	1:30 Z1 to Z2
Total Hrs:			
10:00	1:30	5:15	3:15

WK 22	SW	BIKE	RUN
M		REST DAY	REST DAY
T	#30	Off	1:00 Z2 (at 0:45, insert 5 x 1 min PU @ 1 min Jog)
W		Trans: 0:30 Z2 (QC)	0:15 Z2
R		1:00 Z1 (at 0:45, insert 5 x 1 min PU @ 1 min Spin)	Off
F	0:30 easy	Off	Off
S		0:15 Z1 – easy Bike Safety Check	0:15 Z1 – easy
S	Race	Race (Half Iron-distance)	Race (Half Iron-distance)
Total Hrs:			
4:30 (+Race)	1:15+	1:45 (+Race)	1:30 (+Race)

WK 23	SW	BIKE	RUN
M		REST DAY	REST DAY
T	#31	Off	1:00 Z2
W		Trans: 0:30 Z2 (QC)	0:15 Z2
R		1:00 Z2	Off
F	#32	Off	Off
S		3:45 Z2	Off
S		Off	2:00 Z1 to Z2
Total Hrs:			
10:00	1:30	5:15	3:15

WK 24	SW	BIKE	RUN
M		REST DAY	REST DAY
T	#28	Off	1:00 Z2 (at 0:45, insert 10 min Z4)
W		Trans: 0:30 Z2 (QC)	0:15 Z2
R		1:00 Z2 (at 0:45, insert 10 min Z4)	Off
F	#29	Off	Off
S		3:15 Z2	Off
S		Off	2:30 Z1 to Z2
Total Hrs:			
10:00	1:30	4:45	3:45

WK 25	SW	BIKE	RUN
M		REST DAY	REST DAY
T	#30	Off	1:00 Z2 (at 0:45, insert 10 min Z4)
W		Trans: 0:30 Z2 (QC)	0:15 Z2
R		1:00 Z2 (at 0:40, insert 15 min Z4)	Off
F	#31	Off	Off
S		5:00 Z2	Off
S		Off	0:45 Z1 to Z2
Total Hrs:			
10:00	1:30	6:30	2:00

WK 26	SW	BIKE	RUN
M		REST DAY	REST DAY
T	#32	Off	1:00 Z2 (at 0:40, insert 12.5 min Z4)
W		Trans: 0:45 Z2 (QC)	0:15 Z2
R		1:00 Z2 (at 0:30, insert 20 min Z4)	Off

WK 26	SW	BIKE	RUN
F	#28	Off	Off
S		2:30 Z2	Off
S		Off	3:00 Z1 to Z2
Total Hrs:			
10:00	1:30	4:15	4:15

WK 27	SW	BIKE	RUN
M		REST DAY	REST DAY
T	#29	Off	1:00 Z2 (at 40 min, insert 15 min Z4)
W		Trans: 0:45 Z2 (QC)	0:15 Z2
R		1:00 Z2 (at 0:25, insert 30 min Z4)	Off
F	#30	Off	Off
S		5:00 Z2	Off
S		Off	0:30 Z1 to Z2
Total Hrs:			
10:00	1:30	6:45	1:45

WK 28	SW	BIKE	RUN
M		REST DAY	REST DAY
T	#31	Off	1:00 Z2 (at 0:40, insert 12.5 min Z4)
W		Trans: 0:45 Z2 (QC)	0:15 Z2
R		1:00 Z2 (at 0:35, insert 20 min Z4)	Off
F	#32	Off	Off
S		3:30 Z2	Off
S		Off	2:00 Z1 to Z2
Total Hrs:			
10:00	1:30	5:15	3:15

WK 29	SW	BIKE		RUN
M		REST DAY		REST DAY
T	#28	Off		1:00 Z2 (at 0:45, insert 10 min Z4)
W		Trans: 0:45 Z2 (QC)		0:15 Z2
R		1:00 Z2 (at 0:45, insert 10 min Z4)		Off
F	#29	Off		Off
S		2:00 Z2		Off
S		Off		1:00 Z1 to Z2
Total Hrs:				
7:30	1:30	3:45		2:15

WK 30	SW	BIKE		RUN
M		REST DAY		REST DAY
T	#30	Off		0:45 Z1 (at 0:10, insert 5 x 1 min PU @ 1 min Jog)
W		Trans: 0:30 Z2 (QC)		0:15 Z2
R		0:45 Z1 (at 0:15, insert 5 x 1 min PU @ 1 min Spin)		Off
F	0:30 easy	Off		Off
S		0:15 Z1 – easy Bike Safety Check		0:15 Z1 – easy
S	Race	Race—Iron-distance		Race—Iron-distance
Total Hrs:				
4:00 (+ Race)	1:15+	1:30 (+Race)		1:15 (+Race)

- **Swimming Sessions for the Just Finish Program**

Below are the fifteen swim sessions referred to by number in the swim (SW) column of the training schedules for each of the three phases of the Just Finish Program. The following is an explanation of the abbreviations and terms used:

wu: Warm Up

cd: Cool Down

DR: Swim Drills

Pull: Done with pull buoy (i.e., no kicking).

Pool size: Either yards or meters is fine.

@20sec: Take 20 seconds of rest at the wall after each effort in the set.

Perceived Effort: Warm Up, Cool Down, and Drills should be performed at 65% to 70% perceived effort; Main Sets at 80% to 85% perceived effort.

Base Phase (Weeks 1–10) Swim Sessions (about 1,600 meters/yards)

18. 200wu, 8x50 DR, 5 x 100 @20sec, 8x50 DR, 100 cd

19. 200wu, 8x50 DR, 4 x 125 @20sec, 8x50 DR, 100 cd

20. 200wu, 8x50 DR, 20 x 25 @10 sec, 8x50 DR, 100 cd

21. 200wu, 8x50 DR, 2 x 250 @30sec, 8x50 DR, 100 cd

22. 1,600 straight swim at comfortable pace (75–80% perceived effort)

Build Phase (Weeks 11–20) Swim Sessions (about 2,500 meters/yards)

23. 300wu, 8x50 DR, 8 x 100 @15sec, 8 x 50 @10sec, 8x50 DR, 200 cd

24. 300wu, 8x50 DR, 10 x 75 @20sec, 10 x 50 @15sec, 8x50 DR, 200 cd

25. 300wu, 8x50 DR, 2 x 200 @30sec, 4 x 100 @20sec, 2 x 200 @30sec, 8x50 DR, 200 cd

26. 300wu, 8x50 DR, 25-50-75-100-125-150-175-150-125-100-75-50-25 @20sec, 8x50 DR, 200 cd

27. 2,500 straight swim at comfortable pace (75–80% perceived effort)

Peak Phase (Weeks 21–30) Swim Sessions (about 2,500 meters/yards)

28. 300wu, 8x50 DR, 5 x (100+150) @20sec, 8x50 DR, 200 cd

29. 300wu, 8x50 DR, 6 x 200 @30sec, 8x50 DR, 200 cd

30. 300wu, 8x50 DR, 6 x 75 @20sec, 6 x 125 @10sec, 8x50 DR, 200 cd

31. 300wu, 8x50 DR, 2 x 600 Pull @60sec, 8x50 DR, 200 cd

32. 3,500 straight swim at comfortable pace (75–80% perceived effort)

The Intermediate Program

What if the Competitive Program sounds like too much, but you feel that you can squeeze out a little more weekly training time than is required for the Just Finish Program? What if you don't dream of making it to the awards podium, but you would like to do more than just finish?

The Intermediate Program offers a compromise in time commitment between the Competitive Program and the Just Finish Program. It requires an average of about 10.5 training hours per week over the entire 30 weeks (versus weekly averages of 12 hours and 7 hours, respectively, for the Competitive Program and the Just Finish Program). At its peak the Intermediate Program requires a maximum of 15 hours per week (versus a peak of 20 hours per week for the Competitive Program and 10 hours for the Just Finish Program).

109

Below are each of the three 10-week phases of the Intermediate Program (the Base Phase, the Build Phase, and the Peak Phase). In what follows my comments will be less detailed, since the Intermediate Program is a hybrid of the two programs already presented. If you are interested in this program, please read my full comments on the other two.

- **Base Phase (Weeks 1–10) for the Intermediate Program**

The Base Phase begins with only 6 hours of training in Week 1. There are 2 hours in each sport and eight total workout sessions: three bikes, three runs, and two swims.

From there, training builds by about 1 hour per week for 3 weeks and then decreases by 1 hour every fourth week to allow for greater adaptation (discussed in Chapter 5). By Week 10 we total 11 hours of training spread over eight sessions.

Our Long Bike (discussed in Chapter 3) starts in Week 1 at 1 hour, and builds to 3 hours in Week 10. Meanwhile, our Long Run (discussed in Chapter 3) starts at 45 minutes and increases to 1.5 hours in Week 10.

We will swim two sessions per week, with each session totaling about 2,500 yards/meters.

We have one weekly Transition Session and one weekly 100+ RPM Session (both discussed in Chapter 3).

To sum up, the Base Phase:

- Begins with 6 hours per week and concludes with 11 hours per week;

- Averages about 8.5 hours per week.

The following chart details the Base Phase of the Intermediate Program.

INTERMEDIATE PROGRAM

BASE PHASE: WEEKS 1–10

WK 1	SW	BIKE	RUN
M		REST DAY	REST DAY
T	#33	Off	0:30 Z2
W		Trans: 0:30 Z2 (QC)	0:15 Z2
R	#34	0:30 Z1 (100+ RPM)	Off
F		Off	0:30 Z2
S		1:00 Z2	Off
S		Off	0:45 Z1 to Z2
Total Hrs:			
6:00	2:00	2:00	2:00

WK 2	SW	BIKE	RUN
M		REST DAY	REST DAY
T	#35	Off	0:30 Z2
W		Trans: 0:30 Z2 (QC)	0:15 Z2
R	#36	0:30 Z1 (100+ RPM)	Off
F		Off	0:45 Z2
S		1:30 Z2	Off
S		Off	1:00 Z1 to Z2
Total Hrs:			
7:00	2:00	2:30	2:30

WK 3		BIKE	RUN
M		REST DAY	REST DAY
T	#37	Off	0:45 Z2
W		Trans: 0:30 Z2 (QC)	0:15 Z2
R	#33	0:45 Z1 (100+ RPM)	Off

WK 3			BIKE	RUN
F			Off	1:00 Z2
S			1:45 Z2	Off
S			Off	1:00 Z1 to Z2
Total Hrs:				
8:00	2:00	3:00		3:00

WK 4			BIKE	RUN
M			REST DAY	REST DAY
T	#34		Off	0:30 Z2
W			Trans: 0:30 Z2 (QC)	0:15 Z2
R	#35		0:30 Z1 (100+ RPM)	Off
F			Off	0:45 Z2
S			1:30 Z2	Off
S			Off	1:00 Z1 to Z2
Total Hrs:				
7:00	2:00	2:30		2:30

WK 5			BIKE	RUN
M			REST DAY	REST DAY
T	#36		Off	0:45 Z2
W			Trans: 0:30 Z2 (QC)	0:15 Z2
R	#37		0:45 Z1 (100+ RPM)	Off
F			Off	1:00 Z2
S			1:45 Z2	Off
S			Off	1:00 Z1 to Z2
Total Hrs:				
8:00	2:00	3:00		3:00

WK 6	SW	BIKE	RUN
M		REST DAY	REST DAY
T	#33	Off	1:00 Z2
W		Trans: 0:45 Z2 (QC)	0:15 Z2
R	#34	1:00 Z1 (100+ RPM)	Off
F		Off	1:00 Z2
S		2:00 Z2	Off
S		Off	1:00 Z1 to Z2
Total Hrs:			
9:00	2:00	3:45	3:15

WK 7	SW	BIKE	RUN
M		REST DAY	REST DAY
T	#35	Off	1:00 Z2
W		Trans: 0:45 Z2 (QC)	0:15 Z2
R	#36	1:00 Z1 (100+ RPM)	Off
F		Off	1:15 Z2
S		2:30 Z2	Off
S		Off	1:15 Z1 to Z2
Total Hrs:			
10:00	2:00	4:15	3:45

WK 8	SW	BIKE	RUN
M		REST DAY	REST DAY
T	#37	Off	1:00 Z2
W		Trans: 0:45 Z2 (QC)	0:15 Z2
R	#33	1:00 Z1 (100+ RPM)	Off
F		Off	1:00 Z2
S		2:00 Z2	Off
S		Off	1:00 Z1 to Z2
Total Hrs:			
9:00	2:00	3:45	3:15

WK 9	SW	BIKE	RUN
M		REST DAY	REST DAY
T	#34	Off	1:00 Z2
W		Trans: 0:45 Z2 (QC)	0:15 Z2
R	#35	1:00 Z1 (100+ RPM)	Off
F		Off	1:00 Z2
S		2:45 Z2	Off
S		Off	1:15 Z1 to Z2
Total Hrs:			
10:00	2:00	4:30	3:30

WK 10	SW	BIKE	RUN
M		REST DAY	REST DAY
T	#36	Off	1:00 Z2
W		Trans: 0:45 Z2 (QC)	0:30 Z2
R	#37	1:15 Z1 (100+ RPM)	Off
F		Off	1:00 Z2
S		3:00 Z2	Off
S		Off	1:30 Z1 to Z2
Total Hrs:			
11:00	2:00	5:00	4:00

- **Build Phase (Weeks 11–20) for the Intermediate Program**

The Build Phase begins with about 11 hours of training in Week 11 and then builds to about 12.5 hours in Week 19.

The number of swim sessions per week increases to three and the length of the sessions increases from about 2,500 yards/meters, to about 3,000 yards/meters.

Our Long Bike increases to 4 hours, while our Long Run builds to 2 hours.

We gradually begin to include High Intensity Z4 sessions (discussed in Chapter 6) in both the run and the bike. In Week 12 these Z4 portions total only 15 minutes, or about 2.5% of our total cycling and running. This portion gradually increases each week, and in Week 17 reaches 63 minutes, or about 8% of our total cycling and running.

In Week 18, we have our first practice race (discussed in Chapter 10). It is suggested that this be an Olympic-distance triathlon (1.5K swim, 40K bike, and 10K run). If a race of this distance is not available, you should find a race as close in distance as possible. Chapter 10 has tips on how to locate the right race for you.

Following the race, we have a week of pure aerobic training (Z1 and Z2) to recover and prepare for the work ahead.

To sum up, the Build Phase:

- Begins with about 11 hours per week and concludes with about 12.5 hours per week;

- Averages about 11.5 hours per week.

The following chart details the Build Phase of the Intermediate Program.

INTERMEDIATE PROGRAM

BUILD PHASE: WEEKS 11–20

WK 11	SW	BIKE	RUN
M		REST DAY	REST DAY
T	#38	Off	1:00 Z2 (at 0:10, insert 5 x 1 min PU @ 1 min Jog)
W		Trans: 0:45 Z2 (QC)	0:15 Z2
R	#39	1:00 Z2 (at 0:15, insert 5 x 1 min PU @ 1 min Spin)	Off
F	#40	Off	1:00 Z2 (at 0:45, insert 5 x 1 min PU @ 1 min Jog)

WK 11	SW	BIKE	RUN
S		2:30 Z2	Off
S		Off	1:15 Z1 to Z2
Total Hrs:			
10:45	3:00	4:15	3:30

WK 12	SW	BIKE	RUN
M		REST DAY	REST DAY
T	#41	Off	0:45 Z2 (at 0:10, insert 5 min Z4)
W		Trans: 0:45 Z2 (QC)	0:15 Z2
R	#42	1:00 Z2 (at 0:15, insert 5 min Z4)	Off
F	#43	Off	1:00 Z2 (at 0:45, insert 5 min Z4)
S		2:30 Z2	Off
S		Off	1:00 Z1 to Z2
Total Hrs:			
10:15	3:00	4:15	3:00

WK 13	SW	BIKE	RUN
M		REST DAY	REST DAY
T	#38	Off	0:45 Z2 (at 0:10, insert 3 x 3 min Z4 @ 1 min Jog)
W		Trans: 0:45 Z2 (QC)	0:15 Z2
R	#39	1:00 Z2 (at 0:15, insert 2 x 5 min Z4 @ 3 min Spin)	Off
F	#40	Off	1:00 Z2 (at 0:45, insert 5 min Z4)

WK 13	SW	BIKE	RUN
S		3:00 Z2 (at 2:50, insert 5 min Z4)	Off
S		Off	1:15 Z1 to Z2
Total Hrs:			
11:00	3:00	4:45	3:15

WK 14	SW	BIKE	RUN
M		REST DAY	REST DAY
T	#41	Off	1:00 Z2 (at 0:10, insert 2 x 4.5 min Z4 @ 1.5 min Jog)
W		Trans: 0:45 Z2 (QC)	0:15 Z2
R	#42	1:00 Z2 (at 15 min, insert 3 x 5 min Z4 @ 3 min Spin)	Off
F	#43	Off	1:00 Z2 (at 0:45, insert 7.5 min Z4)
S		3:30 Z2 (at 3:20, insert 5 min Z4)	Off
S		Off	1:15 Z1 to Z2
Total Hrs:			
11:45	3:00	5:15	3:30

WK 15	SW	BIKE	RUN
M		REST DAY	REST DAY
T	#38	Off	1:00 Z2 (at 10 min, insert 2 x 6 min Z4 @ 2 min Jog)
W		Trans: 0:45 Z2 (QC)	0:15 Z2
R	#39	1:00 Z2 (at 15 min, insert 4 x 5 min Z4 @ 3 min Spin)	Off

WK 15	SW	BIKE	RUN
F	#40	Off	1:00 Z2 (at 45 min, insert 7.5 min Z4)
S		4:00 Z2 (at 3:50, insert 5 min Z4)	Off
S		Off	1:30 Z1 to Z2
Total Hrs:			
12:30	3:00	5:45	3:45

WK 16	SW	BIKE	RUN
M		REST DAY	REST DAY
T	#41	Off	1:00 Z2 (at 0:10, insert 5 x 3 min Z4 @ 1 min Jog)
W		Trans: 0:45 Z2 (QC)	0:15 Z2
R	#42	1:00 Z2 (at 0:15, insert 5 x 5 min Z4 @ 3 min Spin)	Off
F	#43	Off	1:00 Z2 (at 0:45, insert 10 min Z4)
S		3:00 Z2 (at 2:50, insert 5 min Z4)	Off
S		Off	1:30 Z1 to Z2
Total Hrs:			
11:30	3:00	4:45	3:45

WK 17	SW	BIKE	RUN
M		REST DAY	REST DAY
T	#38	Off	1:00 Z2 (at 0:10, insert 3 x 6 min Z4 @ 2 min Jog)
W		Trans: 0:45 Z2 (QC)	0:15 Z2

WK 17	SW	BIKE	RUN
R	#39	1:00 Z2 (at 0:10, insert 6 x 5 min Z4 @ 3 min Spin)	Off
F	#40	Off	1:00 Z2 (at 0:45, insert 10 min Z4)
S		3:30 Z2 (at 3:20, insert 5 min Z4)	Off
S		Off	1:15 Z1 to Z2
Total Hrs:			
11:45	3:00	5:15	3:30

WK 18	SW	BIKE	RUN
M		REST DAY	REST DAY
T	#41	Off	1:00 Z2 (at 0:10, insert 5 x 1 min PU @ 1 min Jog)
W		Trans: 0:45 Z2 (QC)	0:15 Z2
R	0:30 easy	1:00 Z1 (at 0:15, insert 5 x 1 min PU @ 1 min Spin)	Off
F		Off	0:40 Z1 (at 0:10, insert 5 x 1 min PU @ 1 min Jog)
S		0:15 Z1 – easy Bike Safety Check	0:20 Z1 – easy PU
S	Race	Race (Olympic distance) Optional: 2:00 hr Z1 – easy (in p.m.)	Race (Olympic distance)
Total Hrs:			
7:45 (+Race)	1:30+R	4:00 (+Race)	2:15 (+Race)

119

WK 19	SW	BIKE	RUN
M		REST DAY	REST DAY
T	#42	Off	1:00 Z1 to Z2
W		Trans: 0:45 Z2 (QC)	0:15 Z2
R	#43	1:00 Z2	Off
F	#38	Off	1:00 Z2
S		4:00 Z2	Off
S		Off	1:30 Z1 to Z2
Total Hrs:			
12:30	3:00	5:45	3:45

WK 20	SW	BIKE	RUN
M		REST DAY	REST DAY
T	#39	Off	1:00 Z2 (at 0:10, insert 4 x 4.5 min Z4 @ 1.5 min Jog)
W		Trans: 0:45 Z2 (QC)	0:15 Z2
R	#40	1:00 Z2 (at 0:10, insert 8 x 4 min Z4 @ 2 min Spin)	Off
F	#41	Off	1:00 Z2 (at 0:45, insert 10 min Z4)
S		4:00 Z2 (at 3:45, insert 5 min Z4)	Off
S		Off	2:00 Z1 to Z2
Total Hrs:			
12:00	3:00	5:45	3:15

- **Peak Phase (Weeks 21–30) for the Intermediate Program**

This phase begins with a Half Iron-distance triathlon (1.2-mile swim, 56-mile bike, and 13.1-mile run), our final practice race. We then enter the key 5-week intensive training volume build-up before the final 3-week pre-race taper and, of course, the Iron-distance race itself.

Weekly training durations start at about 13 hours in Week 21 and gradually increase to 15 hours in Week 25. We remain at 15 hours for 3 weeks, through Week 27. We then drop to about 13 hours in Week 28; 10 hours in Week 29; and 5 hours in Week 30, not including our race.

We continue with three swim sessions per week, but we increase from about 3,000 yards/meters to about 3,500 yards/meters.

Our Long Bike session builds to a maximum of 5.5 hours. Our Long Run increases to a peak of 3 hours.

The High Intensity Z4 portion of our cycling and running starts out in Week 21 at 56 minutes, or about 7% of our volume. In Week 27 we reach our greatest amount of Z4 work: 77 minutes, or about 9% of our total volume.

To sum up, the Peak Phase:

- Begins with about 13 hours per week and peaks at 15 hours per week;

- Averages about 13 hours per week.

The following chart details the Peak Phase of the Intermediate Program.

INTERMEDIATE PROGRAM

PEAK PHASE: WEEKS 21–30

WK 21	SW	BIKE	RUN
M		REST DAY	REST DAY
T	#44	Off	1:00 Z2 (at 0:10, insert 3 x 6 min Z4 @ 2 min Jog)
W		Trans: 0:45 Z2 (QC)	0:15 Z2
R	#45	1:00 Z2 (at 0:15, insert 4 x 7 min Z4 @ 4 min Spin)	Off
F	#46	Off	1:00 Z2 (at 0:45, insert 10 min Z4)

WK 21	SW	BIKE	RUN
S		4:00 Z2	Off
S		Off	1:45 Z1 to Z2
Total Hrs:			
12:45	3:00	5:45	4:00

WK 22	SW	BIKE	RUN
M		REST DAY	REST DAY
T	#47	Off	1:00 Z2 (at 0:10, insert 5 x 1 min PU @ 1 min Jog)
W		Trans: 0:45 Z2 (QC)	0:15 Z2
R	0:30 easy	1:00 Z1 (at 0:15, insert 5 x 1 min PU @ 1 min Spin)	Off
F		Off	0:40 Z1 (at 0:10, insert 5 x 1 min PU @ 1 min Jog)
S		0:15 Z1 – easy Bike Safety Check	0:20 Z1 – easy
S	Race	Race (Half Iron-distance)	Race (Half Iron-distance)
Total Hrs:			
6:15 (+Race)	2:00	2:00 (+Race)	2:15 (+Race)

WK 23	SW	BIKE	RUN
M		REST DAY	REST DAY
T	#48	Off	1:00 Z1 to Z2
W		Trans: 0:45 Z2 (QC)	0:15 Z2
R	#49	1:00 Z2	Off
F	#44	Off	1:00 Z2
S		5:00 Z2	Off
S		Off	2:00 Z1 to Z2
Total Hrs:			
14:00	3:00	6:45	4:15

WK 24	SW	BIKE	RUN
M		REST DAY	REST DAY
T	#45	Off	1:00 Z2 (at 0:10, insert 3 x 6 min Z4 @ 2 min Jog)
W		Trans: 0:45 Z2 (QC)	0:15 Z2
R	#46	1:00 Z2 (at 0:40, insert 15 min Z4)	Off
F	#47	Off	1:00 Z2 (at 0:45, insert 10 min Z4)
S		5:00 Z2 (at 4:45, insert 7.5 min Z4)	Off
S		Off	2:15 Z1 to Z2
Total Hrs:			
14:15	3:00	6:45	4:30

WK 25	SW	BIKE	RUN
M		REST DAY	REST DAY
T	#48	Off	1:00 Z2 (at 0:10, insert 8 x 3 min Z4 @ 1 min Jog)
W		Trans: 0:45 Z2 (QC)	0:15 Z2
R	#49	1:00 Z2 (at 0:35, insert 20 min Z4)	Off
F	#44	Off	1:00 Z2 (at 0:45, insert 10 min Z4)
S		5:30 Z2 (at 5:15, insert 10 min Z4)	Off
S		Off	2:30 Z1 to Z2
Total Hrs:			
15:00	3:00	7:15	4:45

WK 26	SW	BIKE	RUN
M		REST DAY	REST DAY
T	#45	Off	1:00 Z2 (at 0:10, insert 5 x 6 min Z4 @ 2 min Jog)
W		Trans: 0:45 Z2 (QC)	0:15 Z2
R	#46	1:00 Z2 (at 0:30, insert 25 min Z4)	Off
F	#47	Off	1:00 Z2 (at 0:40, insert 12 min Z4)
S		5:30 Z2 (at 5:10, insert 12.5 min Z4)	Off
S		Off	2:30 Z1 to Z2
Total Hrs:			
15:00	3:00	7:15	4:45

WK 27	SW	BIKE	RUN
M		REST DAY	REST DAY
T	#48	Off	1:00 Z2 (at 0:10, insert 10 x 3 min Z4 @ 1 min Jog)
W		Trans: 0:45 Z2 (QC)	0:15 Z2
R	#49	1:00 Z2 (at 0:25, insert 30 min Z4)	Off
F	#44	Off	1:00 Z2 (at 0:40, insert 12 min Z4)
S		5:00 Z2 (at 4:40, insert 15 min Z4)	Off
S		Off	3:00 Z1 to Z2
Total Hrs:			
15:00	3:00	6:45	5:15

WK 28	SW	BIKE	RUN
M		REST DAY	REST DAY
T	#45	Off	0:45 Z2 (at 0:10, insert 3 x 6 min Z4 @ 2 min Jog)
W		Trans: 0:45 Z2 (QC)	0:15 Z2
R	#46	1:00 Z2 (at 0:40, insert 15 min Z4)	Off
F	#47	Off	1:00 Z2 (at 0:40, insert 10 min Z4)
S		4:00 Z2 (at 3:40, insert 12.5 min Z4)	Off
S		Off	2:00 Z1 to Z2
Total Hrs:			
12:45	3:00	5:45	4:00

WK 29	SW	BIKE	RUN
M		REST DAY	REST DAY
T	#48	Off	0:45 Z2 (at 0:10, insert 2 x 6 min Z4 @ 2 min Jog)
W		Trans: 0:45 Z2 (QC)	0:15 Z2
R	#49	1:00 Z2 (at 0:45, insert 10 min Z4)	Off
F	#44	Off	0:45 Z2 (at 0:30, insert 7.5 min Z4)
S		Trans: 2:00 Z2 (QC)	0:30 Z2
S		Off	1:00 Z1 to Z2
Total Hrs:			
10:00	3:00	3:45	3:15

WK 30	SW	BIKE	RUN
M		REST DAY	REST DAY
T	#45	Off	0:45 Z2 (at 0:10, insert 5 x 1 min PU @ 1 min jog)
W		Trans: 0:45 Z2 (QC)	0:15 Z2
R	0:30 easy	1:00 Z1 (at 0:15 insert 5 x 1 min PU @ 1 min Spin)	Off
F		Off	0:40 Z1 (at 0:10, insert 5 x 1 min PU @ 1 min Jog)
S		0:15 Z1 – easy Bike Safety Check	0:20 Z1 – easy (in a.m.)
S	Race	Race—Iron-distance	Race—Iron-distance
Total Hrs:			
5:30 (+Race)	1:30+R	2:00 (+Race)	2:00 (+Race)

- ### Swimming Sessions: Intermediate Program

Below are the seventeen swim sessions referred to by number in the swim (SW) column of the training schedules for each of the three phases of the Intermediate Program. The following is an explanation of the abbreviations and terms used:

wu: Warm Up

cd: Cool Down

DR: Swim Drills

Pull: Done with pull buoy (i.e., no kicking).

Pool size: Either yards or meters is fine.

@20sec: Take 20 seconds of rest at the wall after each effort in the set.

Perceived Effort: Warm Up, Cool Down, and Drills should be performed at 65% to 70% perceived effort; Main Sets at 80% to 85% perceived effort.

Base Phase (Weeks 1–10) Swim Sessions (about 2,500 meters/yards)

33. 300wu, 8x50 DR, 12 x 100 @20sec, 8x50 DR, 200 cd

34. 300wu, 8x50 DR, 4 x 125 @20sec, 4 x 175 @30sec, 4 x 125 @20sec, 8x50 DR, 200 cd

35. 300wu, 8x50 DR, 16 x 25 @10 sec, 1 x 400 @60sec, 16 x 25 @ 10 sec, 8x50 DR, 200 cd

36. 300wu, 8x50 DR, 1 x 300 @40sec, 3 x 200 @30sec, 1 x 300 @30sec, 8x50 DR, 200 cd

37. 2,500 straight swim at comfortable pace (75–80% perceived effort)

Build Phase (Weeks 11–20) Swim Sessions (about 3,000 meters/yards)

38. 500wu, 8x50 DR, 4 x 200 @20sec, 6 x 100 @15sec, 3 x 50 @10sec, 8x50 DR, 300 cd

39. 500 wu, 8x50 DR, 16 x 25 @10sec, 600 Pull, 16 x 25 @10 sec, 8x50 DR, 300 cd

40. 500wu, 8x50 DR, 10 x 50 @15sec, 5 x 100 @20sec, 8 x 50 @15sec, 8x50 DR, 300 cd

41. 500wu, 8x50 DR, 200-300-400-500 @45sec, 8x50 DR, 300 cd

42. 500wu, 8x50 DR, 7 x 125 @20sec, 7 x 75 @15sec, 8x50 DR, 300 cd

43. 3,000 straight swim at comfortable pace (75–80% perceived effort)

Peak Phase (Weeks 21–30) Swim Sessions (about 3,500 meters/yards):

44. 500 wu, 8x50 DR, 12 x 75 @20sec, 12 x 50 @15sec, 12 x 25 @10sec, 8x50 DR, 300 cd

45. 500 wu, 8x50 DR, 5 x 400 @45sec, 8x50 DR, 300 cd

46. 500 wu, 8x50 DR, 6 x (50+100+150) @20sec, 8x50 DR, 300 cd

47. 500 wu, 8x50 DR, 5 x 200 @30sec, 5 x 100 @20sec, 5 x 50 @10sec, 8x50 DR, 300 cd

48. 500 wu, 8x50 DR, 3 x 150 @20sec, 4 x 250 @30sec, 3 x 150 @20sec, 8x50 DR, 300 cd

49. 3,500 Straight swim at comfortable pace (75–80% perceived effort)

CHAPTER 8

Flexibility and Strength Training

Stretching and Warm-Up

This may come as a surprise, but I am not a big believer in a great deal of stretching as part of your warm-up. Light stretching after your training session can be helpful, but I am much more interested in warming muscles up before a workout than in stretching them.

There are many old-school athletes who do their stretching routine in the driveway before their early morning run and then pop right into their training pace. This is not what your muscles need to prepare them for the work ahead, and in fact this type of routine can lead to injury.

The best approach is to warm up your muscles. Begin by walking for 5 to 10 minutes. Then ease into an easy jog and gradually build your pace up to your training pace over a few minutes. Likewise, in a cycling workout, spin easy for 5 to 10 minutes and then gradually build up to your training pace over several minutes. The same also holds true for swimming. All of the swim workouts should include both an easy warm-up and a cool-down period.

The best time for some light stretching is after your workout, as part of your cool-down.

AN *IRONFIT* MOMENT

Meg Waldron on Stretching

As a certified neuromuscular therapist and fitness trainer specializing in post-rehabilitation, Meg Waldron is eminently qualified to advise athletes on stretching. She has worked extensively throughout the country with Nike running camps, the USA Olympic Development Team, as well as with American and international Olympians and hopefuls. Her work combines massage, stretching, and core stabilization exercises to help athletes reach optimum performance. A Philadelphia resident, Meg is a two-time high school track All-American. I was fortunate to meet Meg early on in my triathlon career. Her sensible, time-efficient, and effective approach to stretching has helped me and countless other athletes to both improve performance and reduce susceptibility to injuries. In the following section, Meg shares her approach and provides her stretching program for triathletes, as well as a "short program," for those days when time management is crucial.

Stretching has long been relegated to that thing you do if: (1.) you're already injured; (2.) you think you're getting injured; or (3.) you're nervous at a race and have a few minutes to kill. More and more the act of stretching is coming out of the closet as a viable and shameless way to prevent injury, speed recovery, and improve performance. According to the bulk of evidence, stretching is here to stay and can be that secret weapon when you hit the tri course. But what you do and how you do it makes all the difference in the world.

The three main types of stretching are static, active, and dynamic. Simply put, static stretching is when you hold the stretch position for at least 20 seconds, like yoga. Dynamic stretching is when you use muscle and momentum to swing your trunk, arms, or legs around to loosen them up. Active stretching is when you contract muscles on one side of a joint, like the quadriceps (front thigh), to stretch the muscles on the other side, the hamstring (rear thigh). Oftentimes when you see people using a rope to pull their leg in a stretch position, they are doing active stretching. For example, if you lie on your back and lift your leg straight up using the muscles of the quadriceps, you actively stretch the muscles of the hamstring. Lightly pulling on a rope wrapped around the foot of the stretched leg brings you into a deeper hamstring stretch. Active stretching is particularly well-suited for triathletes for a number of reasons.

Stretches specifically pinpoint the area needing to be stretched, which training and competing athletes need. For example, in the popular routine called Active-Isolated Stretching, there are 3 stretches for the calf, not one. Also, muscles are put in the optimum position to be stretched, so there is less chance of injury from over-stretching.

The academic jury's still out on which is best; however, many athletes have had a tremendous amount of success with active-isolated stretching since its debut at the 1988 Olympic Track Trials.

Active-isolated (AI) stretching works on the evidence that all muscles have an inherent "stretch reflex" that's activated after a strong, rapid movement (like pitching a ball) or after two seconds in a held position (like static stretching). This reflex causes the muscle to begin contracting to protect it from being overstretched or torn. If you keep stretching when the muscle is contracting, you're basically engaging your muscles in a tug of war. The body doesn't like this and will fight you. In AI stretching, you hold each position for only 2 seconds (about the length of an exhale), and then return to the starting position, relax, and repeat. In this way, the muscles are not triggered to contract, thereby providing the best environment for your muscles to do what you want them to do—lengthen. By contracting the opposite muscle group and using a rope to assist with the stretch position, each repetition brings you into a deeper, safer, and more specific stretch than most methods.

The best results come from consistent, gentle stretching that builds upon a daily practice. Once you get your routine down, remember to breathe and relax as you stretch. Keep in mind this important thought: stretching is not about how far you can go, it's about letting go.

Here are two routines you can incorporate into your training. The first is a long program after tough workouts and when you have the time. The second is a short program for the time crunch. If time is really sparse, just do 4–6 reps of each stretch.

- **The Stretches**

  Get a length of dock rope, webbing (like climbers use), or a dog leash and follow these steps in performing each stretch:

  - Contract the muscle group opposite the area you're stretching.

  - Bring each stretch to the point of light irritation.

  - Hold for the length of an exhale (2 seconds). Return to your starting position and relax for 2 seconds. Repeat the stretch.

- **Long Program**

  1. **Hamstring (rear thigh):** Lie on back with right leg bent. Wrap rope around arch of left foot, lock knee and lift straight leg upward, contracting the quads (muscles on the front of the thigh) while you gently assist with rope. Return leg to floor and repeat. Then perform same stretch on opposite side.

  2. **Inner thigh:** Lie on back with legs extended and wrap rope around arch of left foot, then bring the two lengths of rope together and wrap around inside and back of ankle. Point left foot inward and lift leg to the side by contracting outer-thigh and hip muscles. Assist with rope, pulling toward shoulder. Return to original position and repeat. Perform same stretch on opposite side.

  3. **Hip:** Lie on back with legs extended. Wrap rope around arch of right foot, then bring the two lengths of rope together around outside and back of ankle. Point toes of both feet to the right. Bring right leg across opposite leg by contracting inner-thigh muscles. Assist with rope. Return to original position and repeat. Perform same stretch on opposite side.

  4. **Quads (front thigh):** Lie on left side and bring both knees to chest; with left hand, grasp left foot from the outside. With right hand, grasp right ankle and extend right thigh back by contracting gluteus (buttocks) and hamstring muscles and assisting with hand; heel should press into buttocks. Return

right thigh up to chest and repeat. Perform same stretch on opposite side.

5. **Gluteus (buttocks):** Lie on back with right leg extended and pointed inward to stabilize hips. Bend left knee and contract abdominal muscles to lift knee toward the opposite shoulder. Assist with hands on shin and outer thigh. Return to original position and repeat. Perform same stretch on opposite side.

6. **Low back:** Sit with knees bent, legs wide apart and feet flat on the floor and pointing straight ahead. Tuck chin to chest and contract abdominal muscles to bend body toward floor. Assist by placing hands on shins or ankles and pulling forward. Return to original position and repeat.

7. **Mid calf:** Sit with right leg fully extended and left knee bent 90 degrees. Wrap hands around ball of foot. Lift toes toward body by contracting shin muscles and assisting with pull from hands. Repeat. Perform same stretch on opposite side.

8. **Achilles (rear ankle):** Variation of soleus stretch. Sit with right leg extended. Bend left leg, bringing heel to buttocks, and wrap hands around ball of foot. Contract shin muscles to lift toes; assist with hands pulling upward on ball of foot. Repeat. Perform same stretch on opposite side.

9. **Upper calf:** Sit with legs fully extended and about six inches apart. Double up rope and wrap around ball of left foot. Lock left knee and pull toes toward you by contracting shin muscles. Assist with rope. For a deeper stretch, lean forward and allow foot to come off floor when pulled. Repeat. Perform same stretch on opposite side.

10. **Chest (pecs):** Bend your elbow and place your hand behind your head. Step into an open doorway placing the elbow against the face of the doorjamb. Step through the doorway while your elbow gets pulled behind you as it is stopped by the doorjamb. Contract the muscles in the upper back that assist with bringing your arm back further. Repeat. Perform same stretch on opposite side.

11. **Shoulder (rotator cuff):** Bend your elbow at a right angle and press it against your waist. Rotate your hand out to the side and catch it in a doorjamb as you walk through maintaining the right angle. Contract the muscles in the back of your shoulder that further rotate your hand behind you. Repeat. Perform same stretch on opposite side.

12. **Lats (under arms and sides of back):** Stand with your right arm straight overhead. Reach your straightened arm over to the left and grasp right wrist with your left hand. Side bend to the left as you assist the stretch with a pull from your left hand. Repeat. Perform same stretch on opposite side.

13. **Triceps (upper rear arm):** Reach your right arm straight up and then let your hand fall behind your neck. Reach down your back with your hand as you assist the stretch with a gentle push on the elbow from your left hand. Repeat. Perform same stretch on opposite side.

- **Short Program**

  Hamstrings, Quads, Hips, Upper Calves, Pecs, Lats, and Triceps

Strength Training

Is strength training essential to complete an Iron-distance triathlon? No. Is it helpful? Yes, very helpful.

To achieve true overall fitness, strength training is important for virtually everyone. It has great benefits and it complements an overall fitness plan. In addition to building more power for the swim, bike, and run, strength training will help you to achieve greater muscular balance in your body and help to protect against injury.

Strength training becomes increasingly important as we get older, as it helps to slow and even reverse some of the negative effects of aging on our muscles. According to the American Council on Exercise's Personal Trainer Manual, after the age of 25, we lose more than one-half pound of muscle every year.

Given our focus on time-efficient training, we need to make our own decision of whether or not we can afford to dedicate this extra time. While I encourage everyone to regularly complete a strength training program appropriate for them, I can certainly understand that while training for an Iron-distance race, some athletes will need to forgo it due to time constraints. This is doable, and certainly there are many successful Iron-distance triathletes who do not strength train at all.

If you do have to go this route due to time constraints, however, try to make it only a temporary hiatus. Bring strength training back into your overall training program as soon as you can make room for it again.

• Suggested Strength Training Program

Following is a time-efficient strength program developed for Iron-distance triathletes. It is designed to work with my IronFit training programs presented in Chapter 7. This program can usually be completed in about 30 to 45 minutes. So with two strength training sessions per week, you will add about 90 minutes to your training time.

This program utilizes a traditional strength training approach using free weights and/or machines. In the next chapter I will present an exciting new approach to strength training for you to consider. The athlete can select one or the other, or as I will explain in the next chapter, a combination of the two approaches.

Before beginning this (or any other) strength program, please satisfy the following:

1. Be sure to follow the Strength Training Program notes below and consider all the other information in this chapter.

2. Check with your doctor to make sure this program is appropriate for you. As with any exercise program, obtain your doctor's authorization before you even begin.

3. Have a certified personal trainer review the proper technique for each exercise with you, so you can be sure you are training safely. Proper technique is essential for both avoiding injury and maximizing the benefits of your time spent strength training.

STRENGTH TRAINING PROGRAM

EXERCISES	NUMBER OF SETS x NUMBER OF REPETITIONS								
1. Leg Press	1-2 x 12	2 x 12	3 x 10	3 x 10	2 x 8	-	-	2 x 12	2 x 12
2. Lat Pull Down	1-2 x 12	-	3 x 10	-	2 x 8	-	-	-	2 x 12
3. Seated Row	-	2 x 12	-	3 x 10	-	-	-	2 x 12	-
4. Leg Extension	1-2 x 12	2 x 12	3 x 10	3 x 10	2 x 8	-	-	2 x 12	2 x 12
5. Chest Press	1-2 x 12	-	3 x 10	-	2 x 8	-	-	-	2 x 12
6. Chest Fly	-	2 x 12	-	3 x 10	-	-	-	2 x 12	-
7. Leg Curls	1-2 x 12	2 x 12	3 x 10	3 x 10	2 x 8	-	-	2 x 12	2 x 12
8. Biceps Curl	1-2 x 12	2 x 12	3 x 10	3 x 10	2 x 8	-	-	2 x 12	2 x 12
9. Triceps Curl	1-2 x 12	2 x 12	3 x 10	3 x 10	2 x 8	-	-	2 x 12	2 x 12
10. Calf Raises	1-2 x 12	2 x 12	3 x 10	3 x 10	2 x 8	-	-	2 x 12	2 x 12
Number of Weeks	5	5	5	5	8	2	2	4	4
Training Phase:	Base Phase		Build Phase		Peak Phase			Maintenance	

Program Notes:

1. Breathe out to a count of 2 seconds on the "effort" portion of each repetition. Then return the weight to its original position while inhaling to a count of 3 seconds.

2. Choose a weight that you can just make it (with good technique) to the recommended number of repetitions of the first set. It is expected that you will not be able to complete as many repetitions in the second set. For example, if you can just make it to 12 repetitions in the first set, it is likely you will only be able to do a number of repetitions less than 12 in the second set.

3. Rest for 30 seconds after each repetition and between each set.

4. Maintenance Phase: Continue to alternate the two 4-week cycles until your next Base Phase begins.

5. Discontinue Strength Training for two weeks before and two weeks after your Iron-distance race. Also discontinue Strength Training for 5 days before and 3 days after any other races.

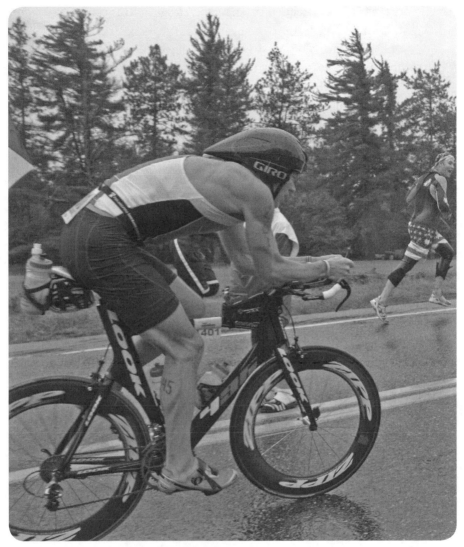

Jeff Kellogg, married, father, business owner . . . Iron-distance triathlete.
Photo Credit: Lynn Kellogg/www.trilifephotos.com.

- **Time-Management Considerations**

    1. **Machines or Free Weights:** The above program suggests strength training machines, instead of free weights. There are pros and cons to each. Free-weight exercises often require more muscle

137

recruitment for needed balance and stability. This can be a plus for triathlon.

While many of the strength training machines do a large amount of the balancing for you, this slight disadvantage is compensated for by a lesser potential for injury, as the machines make it easier to control.

Another advantage of the machines is they usually require less time for set-up before each exercise. Taking weight plates off and on barbells and dumbbells can be time-consuming, versus just moving a pin on the weight deck of a strength training machine. Given our focus on time management (and safe training), these advantages outweigh the disadvantage, so I prefer strength training machines for most athletes training for triathlon. There is risk with all strength training equipment, however, so be sure to have a Certified Personal Trainer familiar with the equipment review each exercise with you and be sure you are using the equipment properly and with good technique.

What if you only have free weights available to you? That is fine. Just be sure to have a Certified Personal Trainer select appropriate substitution exercises for the program above and advise you on proper technique.

2. **Frequency and Timing:** There are many differing opinions on the best number of sessions per week. My suggestion is two, always with at least 48 hours between each. I find that there are only marginal benefits of a third session each week, so from a time-management standpoint, I don't see it to be worth the extra time commitment. Better we put this extra half hour into an area we can derive greater benefit.

It's crucial to be well warmed up before starting strength training. Otherwise, you are risking injury. I suggest a 10 to 15 minute warm up before each strength training session. The best warm-ups include aerobic activities that involve all of your major muscle groups. I prefer power walking on the treadmill for 10 to 15 minutes. A power walk is a steady paced walk with good arm pumping movement. I prefer holding light weights in each hand to help increase the effect.

Here's a time-saving tip: Do your strength training workout immediately after another workout. This way you will already be warmed up. The downside to strength training immediately after other training may be that you are a bit tired, but it's usually a compromise worth making, if it saves you valuable time.

CHAPTER 9

Core and Functional Strength Training

"Do not pray for easy lives.
Pray to be stronger men."

—JFK

Exciting new approaches to traditional strength training have been sweeping the multisports world in recent years. More and more, stability balls and stretch cords are taking the place of barbells and squat racks. The concept of traditional strength training is being replaced by the concept of core and functional strength training.

Traditionally all athletes, including triathletes, would "pump up" with free weights and strength-training machines to help build the strength required for their particular sports activity. Realizing this approach focused mostly on the upper and lower body muscles in isolation, athletes would add sit-ups or crunches to their program to include at least some focus on the abdominal area without integrating the movements of the arms or legs.

For many years this is exactly how my wife Melanie and I approached strength training with our coached athletes. We focused on traditional strength training with free weights and strength-training machines and then added abdominal work in the form of crunches and similar exercises, for what we thought was a more well-rounded program. This began to change, however, as we were introduced to newer core-training techniques many years ago.

By *core strength* we mean the muscles at the center of the body: the abdominal, back, gluteus, and hip-flexor muscles. Not only do these muscles play an important direct role in virtually all triathlon movements, they also serve as stabilizers for the spine, which allow for the proper functioning of and transfer of power to the arms and legs. This inner core strength is where the power begins in all movements.

As Melanie and I moved away from traditional strength training and began a more integrated total body approach, our athletes began to see greater benefits, from injury prevention to increases in power. We began to experience the development of greater functional strength; strength that was more dynamic and applied more directly and specifically to the sports our athletes participated in—the kind of strength required to perform the movements of swimming, running, and cycling.

The reality is that in the sport of triathlon, we never really use either our upper or lower body muscles in isolation. When we use either our upper body or lower body muscles, we engage our core muscles. Each activity—swimming, cycling, and running—is far from isolated. Each requires an amazingly complicated combination of muscle movements orchestrated perfectly throughout our bodies. Knowing this, doesn't it make sense to train this way as well? When we work our upper body muscles, we should perform movements that mirror how we use those same muscles when we perform our sport. Since the core muscles are involved in each triathlon movement, we should also involve them in each movement in our strength training.

There is nothing wrong with the traditional strength-training approach, and for those who prefer it, the strength training program presented in the previous chapter is an excellent complement to any Iron-distance training program. It is absolutely fine if you use one of the IronFit training plans in Chapter 7 and complement it with a traditional strength training program using weights and/or machines. You will achieve your goals. However, for those who want to venture into this newer functional strength approach, this chapter offers the tools to do it.

What Is the Best Strength Training Approach for You?

At this point, you may be saying, "Okay, you gave us the Traditional Strength Training program in Chapter 8 and now you're giving us a two-part Core Strength & Functional Upper & Lower Body Strength approach in this chapter. Which one is best for me?"

I suggest three possible options:

Option One: If you find you prefer the new approach to functional strength and core training, skip the type of traditional strength training program presented in the last chapter and work with both the Functional Core Strength and Functional Upper & Lower Body Strength programs presented in this chapter.

Option Two: For those who prefer the traditional strength training approach, I suggest using the strength training program in Chapter 8, which focuses on the upper and lower body muscle groups and then complement it with the Functional Core Strength Program below. This will add the core elements to traditional strength training for a more complete approach.

Option Three: Use the full Functional Core Strength and Functional Upper & Lower Body Strength programs in this chapter during the competitive season and use the more traditional strength program presented in Chapter 8 with the Functional Core Strength program in the off-season. This provides more variety and flexibility.

The Functional Core Strength Training Programs

Here are two specific strength training programs. The first, **Functional Core Strength**, includes six exercises that focus on the traditional core muscles and utilize the type of exercise equipment usually associated with core training: stability ball, roller, stretch cords, BOSU, medicine ball, and dumbbells.

The second program, **Functional Upper Body & Lower Body Strength**, includes seven exercises that focus on the upper and lower body, just like a more traditional free-weight program, but these exercises include a more functional strength approach and are performed with the same type of exercise equipment used in the Functional Core Strength program: stability ball, stretch cords, dumbbells, etc.

Before beginning this (or any other) strength or core exercise program, please do the following:

1. Follow all the program notes below and consider all the other information in this chapter.

2. Check with your doctor to make sure this program is appropriate for you. As with any exercise program, obtain your doctor's authorization before you begin.

3. Have a certified personal trainer review the proper technique for each exercise with you so you can be sure to train safely. Proper technique is essential for both avoiding injury and maximizing the benefits of your time spent training.

4. Start with the appropriate number of repetitions and sets for your level of fitness or as recommended by your certified personal trainer. One set of ten repetitions is suggested as a starting point for most athletes.

Functional Core Strength Program

- **Exercise One: Front Plank**

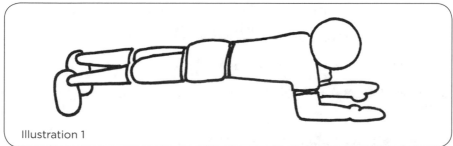

Illustration 1

Description: Lie facedown on a mat or the floor. With your elbows bent under your shoulders and resting on your forearms, lift your torso off the ground, keeping on your toes and forearms. Engage your abdominal muscles to keep your back flat and body in a straight line from your ankles to your head; quads are relaxed. Hold for a count of 30 to 60 seconds (see illustration 1).

Purpose: To build core, hip, and shoulder strength and stability.

First Progression: Same except raise one leg off the ground while maintaining alignment with rest of body.

Advanced Progression: Raise one leg and opposite arm.

143

- **Exercise Two: Side Plank with Arm Raise**

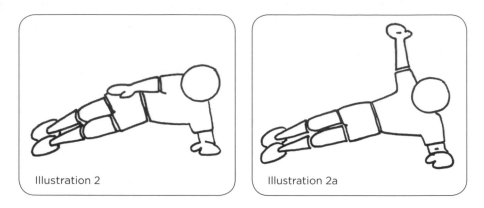

Illustration 2   Illustration 2a

Description: Lie on your side on the floor with your elbow resting directly under your shoulder. Raise your torso off the ground so your body is in a straight line from your ankles to your head. Raise your top arm straight up from your shoulder, palm up and toward the ceiling, hold, and then lower to your side again. Repeat on your other side (see illustrations 2 and 2a).

Purpose: To build core, hip, and shoulder strength and stability.

First Progression: Add a dumbbell in one hand.

Advanced Progression: Raise arm and leg (without dumbbell).

- **Exercise Three: Obliques over BOSU**

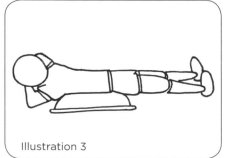
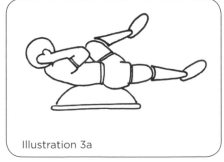

Illustration 3   Illustration 3a

Description: Place the small of your back on the top of the BOSU, hands behind your head; bring your elbow and opposite knee together by engaging your core to raise your torso and knee toward each other. Keep your tongue on the roof of your mouth behind your front teeth to help stabilize your cervical spine and head. The nonactive arm and leg remain in contact with the floor. Repeat on the other side (see illustrations 3 and 3a).

Purpose: To build core strength, stability, and balance.

- **Exercise Four: Ab Crunch with Medicine Ball Raise**

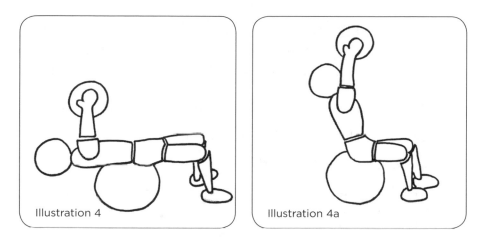

Illustration 4   Illustration 4a

Description: Lie on your back over a stability ball; hold a medicine ball in your hands resting on your chest. Activate your abdominal muscles and raise your torso as you reach the medicine ball toward the ceiling until your arms are straight. Keep your tongue on the roof of your mouth behind your front teeth to help stabilize your cervical spine and head (see illustrations 4 and 4a).

Purpose: To build core strength, stability, and balance.

First Progression: Hold for a count of five.

Advanced Progression: Use weight plate or dumbbells.

- **Exercise Five: Back Extension over Stability Ball**

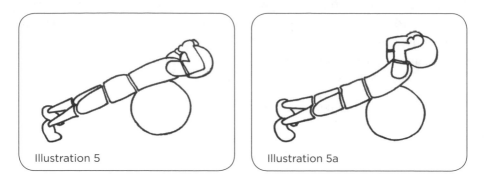

Illustration 5   Illustration 5a

Description: Lie facedown over the stability ball, resting on your midsection, with your legs straight and apart but on your toes, arms locked behind your head. Raise your chest off ball while keeping your head in alignment with your spine (pull chin back). Hold the position, then return to start position and allow your back to relax (see illustrations 5 and 5a).

Purpose: To build lower back strength, stability, and balance.

First Progression: Keep feet together to increase instability on the ball.

Advanced Progression: Use weight plate or medicine ball in hands to increase lower back strength.

- **Exercise Six: Opposite Arm/Opposite Leg on Stability Ball**

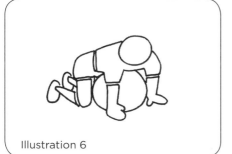
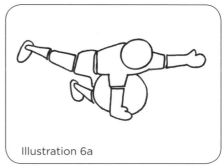

Illustration 6   Illustration 6a

Description: Lie facedown on the stability ball, balancing on your midsection, with legs straight and on toes, hands touching the floor in front. With a straight arm, raise one arm, with thumb up, and opposite leg at the same time. Keep body level over ball and lightly touching hand in front. Hold for three-second count and repeat on other side (see illustrations 6 and 6a).

Purpose: To build lower back strength, stability, and balance.

Functional Upper & Lower Body Strength Program

- **Exercise One: Squat on BOSU with Front Raise Using Dumbbells or Stretch Cords**

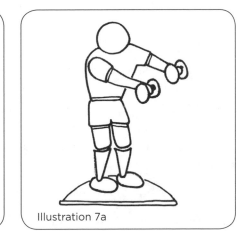

Illustration 7   Illustration 7a

Description: Stand centered on the BOSU while holding light dumbbells or stretch cords at your sides. Sit back into a squat position, leading with your gluteus, and bring quads parallel to the floor (if no previous or current knee issues). As you straighten up from the squat, perform a dumbbell raise (see illustrations 7 and 7a).

Purpose: To build core, hip, glute, and shoulder strength and stability and balance.

First Progression: Stand on the flat side of the BOSU to create instability.

Advanced Progression: Perform a one-leg squat with one foot on floor and then front raise.

- **Exercise Two: Back Lunge with Bicep Curl**

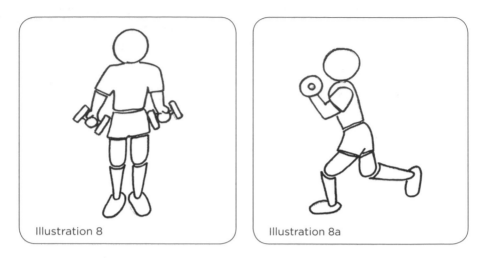

Illustration 8

Illustration 8a

Description: Stand with feet together and light dumbbells at your sides. Perform a back lunge by shifting your weight to your front leg and bending knee while bringing the other leg directly behind you. Hold that position while you perform a bicep curl in both arms. After you finish the curl, bring your back leg next to your front leg and repeat on the other side (see illustrations 8 and 8a).

Purpose: To build glute, quad, hamstring, and arm strength and stability.

First Progression: Standing on a Reebox step, step back off the step into a lunge position.

Advanced Progression: Perform one-leg squat with curl.

- **Exercise Three: One-Leg Squat with Dumbbell Reach & Rotation**

Description: Stand with feet together and a dumbbell in one hand. Raise one leg (with the other knee slightly bent) while holding the dumbbell up in the opposite arm. Perform a one-leg squat and reach the dumbbell across your body toward the planted foot. As you return to the starting position, your arm comes back with extended rotation (see illustrations 9 and 9a).

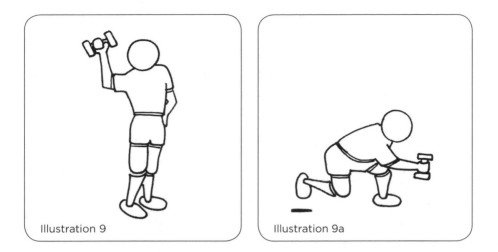

Illustration 9

Illustration 9a

Purpose: To build hip, glute, quadriceps, and shoulder strength and to build stability and balance.

- **Exercise Four: Pullover**

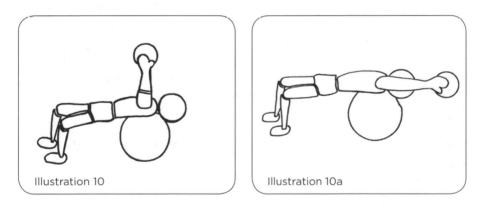

Illustration 10

Illustration 10a

Description: Lie on your back on a stability ball with a medicine ball in your hands; position your feet a little wider than shoulder width and extend your arms toward the ceiling from the shoulders. Bring your arms overhead and parallel to the floor, or to comfortable range of motion. Using your abdominals and lats (latissimus dorsi), pull the medicine ball back over your head above your shoulders (see illustrations 10 and 10a).

Purpose: To build core, chest, back, and shoulder strength.

First Progression: Use one or two dumbbells to perform pullover.

Advanced Progression: Create instability by placing feet together on the center of a BOSU while performing the pullover.

- **Exercise Five: Pushup with Knee Tuck**

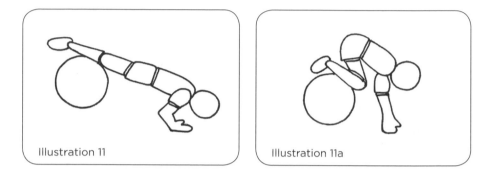

Illustration 11   Illustration 11a

Description: Lie in a pushup position, with your shins on top of a stability ball. Perform a pushup by bending your elbows, bringing your chest to the floor and keeping your head in alignment with your spine. When you get to the top of the pushup, keep your arms straight, engage your abdominal muscles, pull your knees toward your chest, hold, and then return to starting position with arms straight. Repeat pushup and then knee tuck (see illustrations 11 and 11a).

Purpose: To build core, hip, shoulder, arms, and back strength and increase stability and balance.

First Progression: Perform a pike instead of a knee tuck.

Advanced Progression: Perform pushup, then a one-leg knee tuck.

- **Exercise Six: Rear Deltoid Fly on Stability Ball**

Description: Sitting centered on a stability ball, bring your chest to your knees, holding your abs and glutes tight. Holding a dumbbell in each hand on the outside of each foot, raise your arms out to shoulder height, keeping

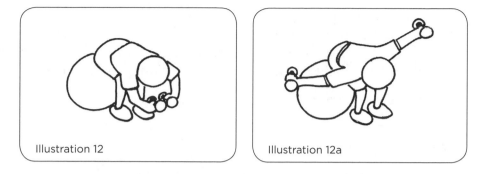

Illustration 12   Illustration 12a

your elbows slightly bent. Use a lighter weight in order to maintain good form. Hold position at the top and then return dumbbells to your sides (see illustrations 12 and 12a).

Purpose: To build shoulder strength and stability.

First Progression: Alternate arms.

Advanced Progression: Stand on one leg.

- **Exercise Seven: Triceps Extension on Stability Ball with One Leg Raised**

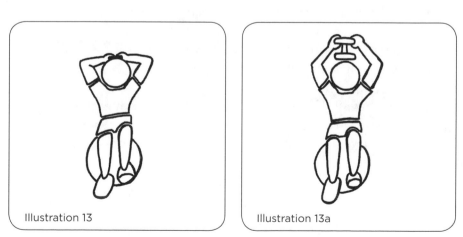

Illustration 13   Illustration 13a

Description: Sit centered on a stability ball with good posture (abdominals engaged, shoulders back, chest out) and a light dumbbell in hands held with bent arms behind your head. Then, while maintaining good posture, tuck your pelvis and raise one leg straight out. Raise the dumbbell toward the ceiling as you extend your triceps without locking your elbows. Hold, and then return to the start position, but keep one leg off the ground. Repeat on the other side with the opposite leg raised (see illustrations 13 and 13a).

Purpose: To build core and arm strength, stability, and balance.

Exercise Equipment

Below is a list of suggested equipment to complete the exercises in the Functional Core Strength and Functional Upper & Lower Body Strength programs:

Stability Ball /Swiss Ball: Round inflated ball that should be sized to fit your height. Available in many sizes (35cm, 45cm, 65cm, 75cm, etc.).

BOSU (acronym for Both Sides Utilized): Inflated ball with a flat side and a half-dome side used to develop balance and stability on an uneven and unstable surface.

Medicine Ball: Round weighted ball with a rubberized coating, available in various weights from 1 pound to 20 pounds.

Dumbbells: Available in various coatings from plastic to metal and various weights from 1 pound to up to 50+ pounds.

Stretch Cord: Rubber or plastic cord with handles in various tensions. These items can be purchased at your local fitness/sports equipment store or online at Web sites such as www.performbetter.com.

CHAPTER 10

Preparing with Training Races

"I have met my hero, and he is me."

—*George Sheehan*

No matter what your experience level, training races can have great value in your preparation for the Iron-distance.

I gradually worked my way up to my first Iron-distance triathlon over a couple of years. I had come from a running background, so I had experienced just about every road race distance possible up to a marathon. When I first tried multisport racing, however, I started with small steps. First I experimented with a short duathlon. Then, I tried a sprint-distance triathlon. Next Olympic-distance triathlons. Eventually I worked my way up to a Half Iron-distance and then to my first Iron-distance.

While some athletes start gradually as I did, many do not. They are bitten by the Iron-distance bug and are pretty much ready to shoot right for Kona. I can understand this. The allure of the Iron-distance is great. Many are so motivated by the ultimate challenge that they don't want to spend time preparing with shorter races.

The flaw with this strategy is that there are just too many variables in racing the Iron-distance. When it comes to Iron-distance racing, experience counts for a great deal. Haste often does make waste.

Your first triathlon shouldn't be at the Iron-distance. Even if your goal is the Iron-distance and nothing else, it's best to utilize appropriate training races to prepare. Training races are important steps along the way to reaching your goal. To maximize your chances of success, use training races to build skills, experience, and confidence.

In this chapter, I will explain what the most appropriate types of races are, and how to maximize their benefit as a training tool.

If you are a relative novice at triathlon, I recommend at a minimum you start by racing a sprint-distance triathlon (e.g., .5-mile swim, 15-mile bike, and 3-mile run) or an international-distance triathlon (i.e., .9-mile swim, 25-mile bike, and 6.2-mile run). Learn all you can from this experience. When you feel ready, race a triathlon at the Half Iron-distance. Similarly, learn all you can from this experience.

Even if you are an experienced triathlete and have raced before, you should include training races in your Iron-distance preparation. In the training plans presented in Chapter 7 I suggest the best times to plan these races on your way to the Iron-distance.

In the following sections I explain what you should try to learn from these experiences, how to select the appropriate races, and how to build them into your training program.

Short-Course through Half Iron-Distance Triathlons

I suggest you complete at least two triathlons as part of your preparation for the Iron-distance. This is true even for those who have past race experience.

My 30-week training plans indicated exactly where these races should be scheduled into your IronFit training program. At the end of this section I suggest resources to help locate the right races for you.

There are so many aspects of Iron-distance racing that you can practice with a shorter race. The practice race is an opportunity to test out your pre-race meal; your warm-up and routine on the morning of the race; your equipment and race clothing; your mental preparation and race tactics; and probably most important, fueling and hydration.

I suggest you treat these races as dress rehearsals and execute your plan exactly as you hope to for the Iron-distance. If all goes well, great! You are right on track. If it doesn't go well, still great! The experience and lessons learned will allow you to revise your plans and be better prepared for the big day.

Each practice race is also a great opportunity to test your equipment in actual race conditions. You should never use some piece of equipment or clothing for the first time in an Iron-distance race. Everything should be tested and re-tested in training. The practice races afford one of the best opportunities to do this.

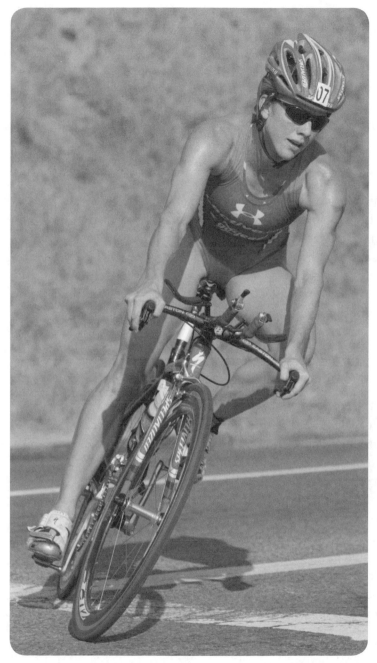

Professional
triathlete and
U.S. Olympic
Triathlon Trials
qualifier Jessi
Stensland.
*Photo Credit:
Action Sports
International.*

Finally, the practice races give you an opportunity to experience the pre-race tension of race morning, and this experience will help prepare you to race well in your Iron-distance race. It's natural to be nervous on race day. What you want to do is channel that anxiety into your performance; you do not want to be numb with fear. Even the world's most experienced triathletes experience butterflies and jitters on race day. Referring to pre-race nerves, two-time World Champion Tim DeBoom once said, "This is what will eventually drive me from the sport." While Tim is affected by pre-race anxiety, he has learned to control his nervousness and channel it into his performance. The experience of racing helps us all to do this.

How can you locate the right races to fit into your Iron-distance training program? There are numerous sources for triathlon information. If you do not know of any local race calendars or similar publications or Web sites, a great place to start is with your country's national governing body for triathlon. In the United States that is USA Triathlon. The organization lists all of its sanctioned races in the United States on its Web site (www.usatriathlon .org). Other great sources are your local bike shop or triathlon club.

Marathons

It's not essential to run a marathon before you attempt the Iron-distance, but for most athletes—and particularly those who do not come from a running background—it can be very helpful. Running a marathon is challenging enough, let alone doing one after a 2.4-mile swim and a 112-mile bike. It's important to have confidence that you can cover the distance. You do not want to doubt your marathon ability. You need to develop a real "been there, done that" confidence in your running. You need to be comfortable with the uncomfortable.

If you have never run a marathon before, I suggest that you do a "practice marathon" at some point prior to your Iron-distance race. Due to the recovery time required after a marathon (a significant interruption in the training cycle), it's important not to schedule a marathon close to your Iron-distance race. Ideally, you should run the marathon prior to beginning your 30-week IronFit training program.

For example, if you were planning on an Iron-distance race in late July, and you were to start your 30-week program in January, then the prior

October through December period would be the best time to schedule your marathon. This way, you could prepare for and complete it prior to your Ironman program. You would begin Iron-distance training with both the physical benefits of marathon training and the confidence of having knocked off this serious endurance challenge.

How can you find the right marathon for you? There are several running magazines and Web sites with information and race schedules. One of my favorite sources is the marathon race calendar on the Web site affiliated with *Runner's World* magazine (www.runnersworld.com). It lists hundreds of U.S. and international marathons.

As you will find, marathons are quite plentiful—on most weekends you can find one or more. The Web site provides contact information for most races and a direct link to the race's Web site.

Century Rides

Have you ever ridden your bike over 100 miles at one time? Like running a marathon, participating in a Century Ride is also a great way to build your confidence. I say "participating" because these are usually organized more as fun rides than as competitions. Some athletes ride them for time, but most do not ride them competitively. This is good for training purposes because it makes them less intimidating and a great way to build your confidence.

Century Rides can also be utilized for your long training rides. If solo rides are not that appealing to you, Century Rides provide company and inspiration. Unlike marathons, which require focused training and then time to recover afterward, Centuries can be built right into your training program. No special preparation is needed, particularly in the final 10-week Peak Phase of your 30-week Ironman program. These rides can just be substituted for one of your scheduled Long Rides.

The best way to find a good Century Ride in your area is to stop in at your local bike shop. Your local bike shop is also the place to find out about local riding clubs and regularly scheduled group training rides in your area.

Other good sources to locate Century Rides include the Ultra Marathon Cycling Association's Web site (www.ultracycling.com), the American Cycling Association's Web site (www.americancycling.org), and USA Cycling's Web site (www.usacycling.org).

Open-Water Swims

Open-water swim races are not necessary for all triathletes, especially those who have successfully completed a shorter distance triathlon. However, for weaker swimmers and those who lack confidence in their swimming, open-water swim races are a great idea. The best way to get over your jitters is to experience open-water swimming on a regular basis.

Convenience is a factor in deciding whether you want to add some open-water swims to your preparation. If participating in these races requires a great deal of travel, it may not be worth it. But if they are available in your area you should consider them.

I am fortunate to live within an hour of the New Jersey shoreline. From June to August, there is an open-water race at one of the many shore towns on almost every weekend. They are usually in the early morning and 1 mile in distance, and sometimes longer. I can usually take part in these races and be home in only a couple hours. These races are so convenient and such a great way to gain open-water race experience that I find them hard to pass up.

How can you locate open-water swim races in your area? You can find schedules and information on open-water swim events on the USA Swimming Web site (www.USASwimming.org), in the Long Distance section of the United States Masters Web site (www.USMS.org/longdist/), and at www.oceanswims.com.

IRONFIT PROFILE

Charles Windus (written in 2004)

Charlie Windus is a top age-group Iron-distance triathlete. He qualified for the Hawaii Ironman World Championships in 1997, 2000, and 2002, and placed well in his age group each time. Charlie has twice won his age group at Ironman Florida, and previously held the Ironman Florida course records for both the 50–54 and 55–59 age groups.

Charlie is married with three children, one of whom recently went off to college, and a dog. He lives in central New Jersey and works as an analytical chemist for GlaxoSmithKline, a major pharmaceutical company. Charlie works 40 to 45 hours per week, plus about 20 minutes each way for commuting. He usually leaves for the office by 7:00 a.m. and returns around 4:00 p.m.

Charlie was immediately attracted by the aura of the Iron-distance, but it took him almost twenty years to get to the point where he felt ready to give it a try; he started in triathlon in his late forties. Starting with shorter races, he gradually moved up to long-course racing. Today he is respected as one of the top triathletes in the world in his age group.

During the week, Charlie does most of his training in the late afternoons; usually he is able to get in 2 hours or more if needed. He does his longer sessions on the weekends, doing his best to plan them around the schedules of his wife and children. Charlie usually swims with a Masters group in the evening, or catches up with swim workouts on the weekends if necessary.

Charlie's family is surprised at how well he does in triathlon. To them, Charlie's investment in his training does not seem so great, given the level of success he has had. Charlie credits a time-efficient training program for his ability to compete well while also attending to the needs of his family and career. Charlie's family is very supportive of his racing; they especially enjoy trips to races in tropical locations like Hawaii and Florida.

Charlie's colleagues at work are also very supportive. They tend to be impressed and inspired by his accomplishments. Some managers have even asked him if he was sure that he was getting enough time to train before major races. They all want him to succeed and admire the way in which he can keep his life in such good balance. They are often curious about how much training he does and how he can fit it all in.

Following are some of Charlie's training and time-management techniques.

Keep Physical Energy Up: Charlie finds this to be challenging while in peak training periods. He feels that his physical freshness follows his mental freshness. If he feels tired or stale, he takes an extra day off to rest. If the tiredness continues, he takes additional days off or does a lighter week of training than originally planned.

Live a Low-Stress Life: Charlie admits that this is easier said than done, but argues that most people can do a great deal to reduce stress if they choose to. For himself, Charlie tries to be more flexible with others and not so quick to correct others' mistakes. By doing so he feels that he greatly reduces his stress and duress.

Be Flexible: Charlie also tries to be flexible in his training. He trains with a plan and tries to stick with it, but when surprises come up he adjusts. He modifies his program when necessary, trying as best he can to fit in as much as possible. If he can't accomplish everything in a session that he set out to, he doesn't obsess about it. He does the best he can and leaves it at that.

Accomplish Two Things at Once: For effective time management, Charlie combines tasks whenever possible. He takes the dog with him on his runs. He combines family vacations with races. He gets caught up on the news while he stretches.

Make Multiple Meals: Instead of spending a great deal of time in the kitchen during peak training periods, Charlie often prepares enough of a dish to furnish a second or even a third meal.

CHAPTER 11

Technique

"Fitness is what happens while you are
practicing good technique."

—Terry Laughlin

Efficient technique is essential to Iron-distance success. When you are
powering your body over 140 miles, you can't afford to waste any energy.
And that's what inefficient technique means: wasted energy. It's as simple as that. We want to become as fit as we possibly can, and then use our
fitness as efficiently as we can.

In this chapter I will help you to improve your swimming, cycling, and
running techniques. I will explain proper technique for each sport, identify
the most common errors, and help you make the needed corrections.

Swimming Technique

As important as technique is in cycling and running, it is even more so in swimming. Water is 800 times denser than air. Most triathletes spend plenty of time
trying to reduce drag when it comes to their bikes, but let me tell you, it's nothing compared to the drag we experience in the water. Being as aerodynamic
(actually, hydrodynamic) as possible is crucial to fast, efficient swimming.

If you have a swimming background, your freestyle swim technique is
probably already pretty good. Freestyle is generally the fastest of the strokes
and is therefore used by virtually all triathletes. Even if you reached only the
high school level as a competitive swimmer, you have a big head start over
most new triathletes.

It will be a bit more challenging for those of us without a swimming
background. As many find, even if you know how to swim and can get from

161

one side of the pool to the other, there is a great deal more to efficient tri-athlon swimming. Below I summarize the primary elements of good Iron-distance swim technique, identify the common errors, and explain how to correct them.

- **Body Position**

While the most attention is usually given to stroke mechanics, I find the greatest area for potential improvement for most adult swimmers is in their body position.

As mentioned, you need to become as hydrodynamic as you possibly can in the water. Water is so dense that every little bit of resistance is greatly multiplied. You want to turn yourself into a sleek, slippery torpedo and slide easily through the water.

Your upper torso should be pressed into the water, allowing your hips and legs to rise to the surface. If your hips and legs hang low and out of the slipstream created by your upper body, you will needlessly increase your profile, and thus increase drag.

You also want to have good body rotation. Body rotation refers to the side-to-side rolling motion associated with technically good swimming. This rolling motion has many advantages. First, it adds leverage to each stroke. Instead of just "muscling" each stroke, you literally get your body into it.

Second, body rotation makes breathing more efficient. With good rota-tion, your head just rotates with the rest of your body, putting your mouth in a position to breathe. By contrast, if you have to lift your head to breathe, you create up-and-down turbulence.

Finally, this side-to-side motion also slightly decreases your body pro-file, thereby reducing your drag in the water.

These are the most common body position flaws:

- **Low Hips:** New swimmers often let their hips and legs hang low in the water, causing significant resistance as the upper body tries to drag them through the water. Check your form to make sure that your upper torso is pressed into the water thereby allowing your hips and legs to rise up and out of the way. They should trail in the slipstream created by your upper body. Your "seat" should actually be high enough that it breaks the surface of the water; it should not hang below the surface.

- **Swimming Flat:** Another common flaw is swimming "flat," with little or no body rotation. This causes a whole host of problems, all of which slow you down. These include not utilizing body leverage and instead just "muscling" your strokes with your arms; inefficient breathing due to poor body rotation and head position; and increased body profile.

The Chest Lean drill, which I introduce in the next section, will help you improve your body position. If you find that you are swimming "flat," the Three Stroke Kick-on-Side drill will help you improve your body rotation.

- **Stroke Mechanics**

Each freestyle stroke includes the following elements: the Entry, the Catch, the Pull, and then the Release/Recovery. We will consider them in order.

The Entry

Your hand should enter the water above your head and in front of your shoulder. You should then extend your hand straight out under the water in the direction you are swimming. As you extend your hand, you should allow your body to roll up on its side and glide through the water.

Common Entry flaws:

- **Overreaching:** Instead of entering in front of the shoulder, the hand crosses over the centerline of the body. This creates a fishtailing effect that slows the swimmer.

- **Limited Glide:** Beginning your stroke immediately, before allowing your arm to extend out and your body to roll up on its side and glide. There needs to be a pause at the end of the extension. When your hand enters the water and slides out forward in the direction you are swimming, it should actually stop momentarily before beginning the Catch. This is where you want to experience a gliding sensation. Swimming is not a constant windmilling motion; it is a series of motions: stroking, rolling side-to-side, and gliding.

The Catch

The next phase of the stroke is the Catch. Your shoulder rolls forward as your elbow bends but remains high in the water. You "catch" the water with your hand and forearm by positioning them as if you are wrapping your hand and forearm around a barrel in the water.

Common Catch flaws:

- **Dropping Elbows:** Not keeping the elbows high in the water, and allowing them to drop. This results in a weak Catch. Your arm should be bending at the elbow and your elbow should remain high in the water. This allows you to "catch" the water with your forearm, thereby giving you a much bigger paddle to stroke with. Instead of just your hands, you are using both your forearms and your hands. One of the most common stroke flaws is a straight-arm style of swimming.

- **Lack of Shoulder Roll:** Not allowing the shoulder to roll forward, thus cutting short the forward extension.

The Fists drill, which I introduce below, will help you to develop an efficient Catch.

The Pull

In the Pull phase, we "pull" the water back in an S-like shape. If you are rotating your body properly this should occur naturally. Your hand will sweep out slightly, then in toward the centerline of your body, and then out again, just below your pelvis. Only the slight outward sweep in the beginning needs to be a conscious movement. The remainder of the S-shape will occur naturally as your body rotates from side to side in the water. Your hand should fully extend past your hip at the end of the stroke.

Common Pull flaw:

- **Lack of Follow-Through:** Pulling the hand out of the water too soon and not following through well. You should allow your arm to follow through completely; your hand should extend down to your upper thigh and exit the water below the bottom of your swimsuit.

The One Arm and Catch-Up drills, which I introduce below, will help you to develop a powerful Pull.

The Release/Recovery

The final phase of the stroke is the Release/Recovery. At the end of the pull, your hand will release the water and your palm will turn inward towards your body. From that point, your arm will gently return through the air until the time it reenters the water in front of your shoulder. The power portion of the stroke occurs underwater. The recovery should be loose and relaxed. I often encourage my swimmers to have a "soft" recovery.

Common Recovery flaw:

- **Muscling the Recovery:** Aggressively muscling the recovery above the water. This is wasted energy. The Recovery should not look like you are throwing a punch. The power part of the stroke is the Pull. This final phase should be relaxed. Your elbow should point skyward, and the hand and forearm should hang relaxed from the elbow.

The Fingertip Drag drill, which I introduce below, will help you to develop a relaxed and efficient Recovery.

- ## The Kick

While a big powerful kick may be desirable in shorter races, I recommend a smaller, more efficient kick for Iron-distance racing. We want to save our legs for the work ahead. After all, we have a 112-mile bike ride and a marathon to deal with. If we can swim fast without relying much on our legs, let's do it.

The kick should help you rotate your body and maintain proper position, but it should do very little to propel you forward. We are going to leave that primarily up to the arms. The main purpose of the kick is to stabilize you in the water and contribute to your body rotation.

Common Kick flaws:

- **Big Kick:** Too large and wide a kick. Many swimmers try to propel themselves through the water with a wide and powerful kick. Again, this is inefficient for longer races. It can throw off your body position, create drag, and waste energy. You want your kick to be small, efficient, and in the slipstream.

- **Too Many Kicks per Stroke:** This is the frequency of the kick, not the size. How often should you kick? Experts differ on this one, but I find a two-beat kick is best for most endurance swimmers. This means one kick for every one stroke. Swimmers who race shorter distances in the pool frequently have a four or six-beat kick. If this is the way you are most comfortable, it may not be worth changing. But if you are just starting out as an adult swimmer, a two-beat kick is the best way to go.

While several of the drills below will help you to develop an efficient kick, the Vertical Kicking drill is particularly beneficial.

- **Turbulence**

I have already mentioned turbulence a couple of times as it is a technique problem that overlaps various areas. By turbulence I mean any action that causes your body to rock up and down or "fishtail" from side to side in the water. Turbulence creates drag, slowing you. Again, you want to be like a slick torpedo sliding through the water, with none of this turbulence. Turbulence will only slow you down and waste energy. Below are the common causes of turbulence.

Side-to-Side Turbulence

One of the most common causes of side-to-side turbulence is crossing over in front of your head with your hand before it enters the water. This causes your body to swivel through the water. You want your left hand to enter the water at 11 o'clock, and your right hand at 1 o'clock. If this is an issue for you, practice your entry.

Kicking "too big," and bringing your feet out of your slipstream, can also cause this fishtailing effect. The Vertical Kicking drill, presented below, will help you develop a tight, efficient kick. In addition, doing all of the drills with short-style fins will improve your kick.

Up-and-Down Turbulence

One of the most common causes of up-and-down turbulence is lifting your head up to breathe. When the head comes up, the lower body goes down to compensate; when the head goes back down, the lower body comes up to compensate. This up-and-down motion slows you in the water.

If you find that you do this, focus on keeping your head lower in the water and, instead of lifting your head to breathe, turn your body and breathe to the side without lifting your head.

• Technique Drills

These are some of the best drills for correcting the most common technique flaws. Select from these drills to make up the drill sets in the 30-week IronFit training programs in Chapter 7. You can work with all of them, but give special focus to those drills that work on the areas in which you need the most improvement, and be sure to focus on that specific aspect while you complete the drills.

I recommend that you use short fins for most drills. They will help you to develop a smaller, tighter kick and will help you to maintain a speed closer to your normal swim speed, otherwise your speed would be too slow during the drills. The bigger fins can have you swimming so much faster than your normal speed that the sensation is unnatural.

1. **Chest Lean:** Wearing fins, kick with your face down, chin pointed to the bottom of the pool and your hands held closely at your sides. These are the key setup points: (a) position your head so that the water breaks on top of your head, not on your forehead; (b) lean on your chest; and (c) raise your hips up to the surface of the water. Your "seat" should actually be slightly above the surface.

When you need to take a breath, lift your head and breathe to the front. When you do this, you will find that your hips and legs will drop down lower in the water. To reestablish your original position, keep your hands at your sides and follow the three points above.

This drill helps to correct poor body position. It teaches you to maintain a low head position in the water, to press down with your upper body, and to bring your hips and legs to the surface. The drill teaches you to maintain this position while swimming without having to think about it. This should be our ultimate aim: to maintain efficient body position automatically.

2. **Three Stroke Kick-on-Side:** Kick with fins while lying on your side on the surface of the water. Your arm on the upside should be held at your side, and your arm on the downside should be extended straight out in the direction you are heading. Your downside shoulder should be pressed against the side of your head. After about ten kicks, take three slow strokes and then assume the same position on the opposite side of your body. After ten more kicks, take three strokes again and assume the same position on the original side. Continue this sequence.

This drill helps to develop good body rotation and glide. As we have seen, efficient swimming is not about staying facedown in the water; we want to have good body roll from side to side as we swim. Swimming flat in the water is a common flaw. By rolling up on your side, you develop better leverage with each stroke and better glide with higher body position.

3. **One Arm:** Wearing fins, swim in the "Superman" position, with your face down and both hands extended out in front of you, pointing in the direction you are traveling. Take one perfect stroke with your left hand (breathe on this stroke) and return to the Superman position for three seconds. Continue this sequence with the same arm for the full length of the pool, and then repeat the same drill with the opposite arm.

This drill provides a great opportunity to focus solely on taking a perfect stroke. You can work on all stroke elements: the Entry, Catch, Pull, and Release/Recovery.

4. **Catch-Ups:** In this drill you wear fins and swim normally except for this: You will hold your hand extended out in front of you and delay taking your next stroke until the other hand catches up and touches the extended hand. Think about delaying each stroke and gliding a little more through the water before taking your next stroke.

    This drill teaches you to glide more with each stroke. A common flaw is to stroke continually, like a paddleboat. This is inefficient. After propelling your body forward, you want to get a great glide before taking your next stroke.

5. **Fists:** This is one of the only drills that should be completed without fins. Swim normally, but with clenched fists instead of open hands. Visualize yourself putting your forearm around a barrel and pulling it behind you. Use your whole forearm as "your paddle."

    This drill helps us to develop a more complete Catch. Instead of just using our hands as paddles, we want our paddle to be the entire area from the fingertips to the elbow. By minimizing the contribution of the hands, this drill helps us develop a better Catch with our forearms.

6. **Fingertip Drag:** In this drill you swim normally, with or without fins, but instead of a high Recovery above the water, keep your hand in contact with the water on the Recovery by dragging your fingertips across the water. Your hand should exit and enter the water in the normal place, but not lose contact with the water in between. Your elbow should be pointed towards the ceiling with your forearm and hand hanging relaxed below.

    This drill develops a relaxed and efficient Recovery. As I mentioned above, many swimmers throw their arm forward aggressively in the Recovery phase, as if they are throwing a punch. This is wasted energy.

7. **Vertical Kicking:** Wearing fins, kick in place in the vertical position, with your head above the surface of the water and the rest of your body directly below you. Focus on having a small, powerful kick as opposed to a wide, spread-out kick. Use your gluteus maximus (seat muscles) and hamstrings to generate the

power while your feet remain relatively close together (six to eight inches apart). I often encourage the swimmers I coach to think of a boxer hitting a speed bag, as opposed to a boxer hitting a body bag, as they do this drill.

Start by doing this drill with your hands held down at your sides. As your kick gets stronger, you can add to the challenge by clasping your hands behind your head. This drill is measured in time, not distance. I suggest starting at 1 minute, and then gradually building it up to 5 minutes over time.

POOL TOYS

By "pool toys" I mean any of the many popular apparatuses used by swimmers as training aids. As mentioned above, I suggest short fins for all but one of the technique drills. Otherwise, I am not a big fan of pool toys for adult swimmers. If you come from a competitive swimming background and you have experience with them, some are fine to use. Otherwise avoid them. They can reinforce bad habits and even cause injury. Following are some of the most common pool toys, and some of the downsides involved in using them.

Kickboards: Unless you have a lot of experience with them, kickboards can reinforce poor body position. They hold the upper body up, and let the lower body sink down—just the opposite of what most swimmers need to do. In addition, they can reinforce a big kick, which I don't recommend for endurance swimming.

Paddles: Unless you are an experienced swimmer, avoid paddles. They are risky for the vast majority of swimmers. If not used correctly, they can be a crutch for a weak Catch (they can have the opposite effect of the Fists drill), and they can be dangerous to your shoulders and can cause injury. Please leave this one alone.

Pull Buoys: This is about the only pool toy I ever use in the Masters swimming program I coach. They can be good for isolating your stroke and developing your power, without the benefit of a kick. However, they can become a crutch for bad body position and a weak kick. So use them in moderation.

Cycling Technique

While technique is everything when it comes to swimming, we can also become faster and more efficient on the bike by employing good technique. In this section I will present proper technique for the key elements of cycling, including pedaling motion, cadence, climbing, descending, and cornering.

- **Pedaling**

In general, you should "spin circles." That is, as much as possible, you should apply even force to the pedals through all points in the pedal revolution. Avoid pushing down and pulling up on the pedals. This is inefficient and may also lead to injuries. This "mashing" of the pedals is a common mistake, especially for athletes coming from a running background.

Use the High RPM Spin sessions and the "90 circles" visualization I discuss in Chapter 3 to help perfect spinning circles.

As for cadence, most of your cycling should be in the range of 80 to 100 revolutions per minute (RPM). When you climb a big hill, it's normal for your cadence to drop to below 80 RPM. While descending or biking with a strong tailwind, your cadence may be up above 100 RPM. And for most cycling in between, your cadence should be around 90 RPM. There is a great deal of disagreement on this topic, and there are plenty of great cyclists who violate these parameters. But for most, I find this range works best.

If your cadence is consistently too high, you are not taking full advantage of your power and you are giving up some speed. If your cadence is too low, you are pushing too large a gear, which means that your cycling form may be inefficient and you may even risk injury. I suggest that you stay within the 80 to 100 RPM cadence range and experiment to find the optimal level for you.

- **Hill Climbing**

Many triathletes fear hills and avoid courses with challenging topography. You can do this and continually search out the flat races, but I recommend that you "befriend the enemy." Meet the challenge of hills head-on, and become a strong climber on your bike. The rewards are great. I often tell my athletes that climbing is what "separates the kids from the grown-ups" in triathlon.

Proper climbing technique is important for Iron-distance racing because we cannot afford to waste energy. Inefficient technique causes you to expend more energy than is necessary and may raise your heart rate above the optimal level. This will come back to haunt you later in the race.

When you climb in the seated position, you want to slide back on your seat slightly and try to engage your powerful upper leg and "seat" muscles.

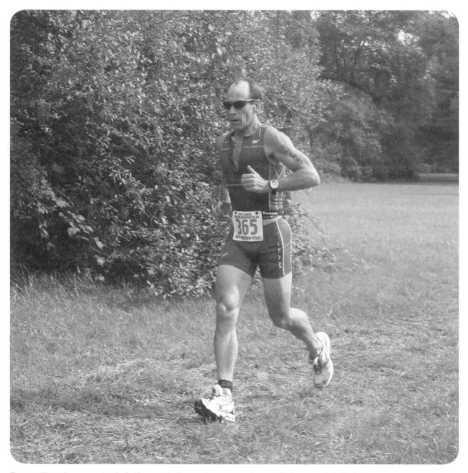

Peter Turek, married, father, civil engineer . . . Iron-distance triathlete.
Photo Credit: Tina Tedford.

When you climb while standing, you want to hold your torso steady as you rock your bike from side to side. You want to keep your wheels in a straight line. This allows you to bring in the powerful hamstring muscles to assist with the propulsion of the bike.

A common mistake is bouncing up and down on the bike to get up the hill in the standing position. This technique is wasteful. Again, you want to stand steady on the bike and rock it from side to side. This leveraging of the upper body can help save your legs and keep your heart rate down.

Another common mistake is allowing your wheels to wander from a straight path up the hill, instead carving an S-shape. The Iron-distance is plenty long enough; you don't want to add to it. The shortest distance between two points is a straight line. You want to cut an imaginary straight line up the hill.

When should you stand and when should you sit? For shorter hills, say up to a half mile, I suggest sitting for the first two-thirds and then shifting up one gear and standing for the final one-third. Don't forget to power right over the top of the hill.

Always plan ahead as you approach a hill. Size it up and have a strategy on how you will cycle it. In general, if your cadence slows to an uncomfortable level—for most cyclists this amounts to a drop in cadence of 10% or more—you need to take action. Either shift gears or stand.

For long steep climbs of a half mile or more, I suggest alternating standing and sitting. Find a time interval that feels comfortable. For instance, you can sit for 1 minute, then click up one gear and stand; after standing for 1 minute, click down a gear and sit for 1 minute. Keep alternating back and forth and adjusting your gearing as you power up and over the hill.

For climbs of a low grade, you are usually better off to stay seated throughout, and only stand occasionally to give your muscles a break.

• Descending Hills

The problem with descending for most triathletes is simple: They are scared. And why shouldn't they be? You are flying down a hill at over 40 mph, with nothing between you and the unforgiving asphalt but a few pounds of carbon fiber.

It's not uncommon to see triathletes nervously feathering their brakes all the way down a hill, particularly when crosswinds are present. This is unfortunate, because fear causes these athletes to give up significant time in their races. Nonetheless, if you do feel unsafe, you should always slow down or even stop, and regain your composure. Safety is always the most important thing.

The key to descending is knowledge and confidence. You need to know how to position yourself safely on your bike, and you need to be confident that your equipment is 100% safe and reliable. You want to be aerodynamic, stable, and safe.

To be safe, you want to put your weight back on the saddle. Get in a low but very stable position. Keep your hands firmly on the handlebars or in your aero bars, and near your brakes. Always take the safest line possible, and keep looking down the hill and planning your line out as far as you can in advance.

As for your equipment, you want to be 100% confident. The only way to achieve this is to use high quality equipment, have it serviced frequently by a qualified professional, and always do a complete bike check before every ride. In the following, I present a ten-point pre-ride safety check used by many of my coached athletes. If you find that you really cannot get comfortable with descending (or with climbing, for that matter), there are plenty of relatively flat and non-technical Ironman courses. There is nothing wrong with choosing one of these races. We will discuss race selection in Chapter 16.

TEN-POINT BIKE SAFETY CHECK

A significant number of athletes experience bike mechanical problems in races. These problems cost them valuable time, or worse, even injury. It's frustrating to train so hard and make such great sacrifices for a race, only to have it end this way.

The good news is that while we cannot eliminate every potential bike problem, even a basic pre-race bike check can go a long way toward heading off these problems. I recommend that athletes perform a bike safety check every time they head out for a ride, and a specific pre-race bike check the day before every competition.

While this is always important, it is especially important if you are traveling to a race. Your bike can easily be damaged during transport, sometimes in such a minor way that you will not even notice—until mile 2 in the race! If you are flying to a race and need to reassemble your bike upon arriving, there is the additional risk of error when you put it back together.

You should do a thorough check of your bike and cycling equipment early in the day before the race. Don't wait until the late afternoon bike check-in; you may need time to get to a bike shop if repairs are needed.

Following is a quick and easy ten-point pre-race bike equipment check that will help you stay safe and avoid some of those time-wasting problems that can occur on the racecourse.

1. **Tires:** Flat tires are probably the most common bike problem. Slowly spin the wheels and check your tires closely for imbedded debris, cracks, or worn spots. If you see anything that looks questionable, put on a new tire and test it out before the race. Under- and over-inflated tires should also be avoided. Know the correct inflation level for your tires and always check them before every ride.

2. **Wheels:** Wheels can easily be damaged when transporting the bike to the race. A wheel even slightly out of true can cause big problems. Check each of your spokes for tightness, if you are using spoked wheels. Raise each wheel off the ground and spin it gently. Watch closely for wobbliness. If your wheel is out of true, head for the bike shop; this is something that needs to be fixed with special equipment.

3. **Brakes:** Spin each wheel gently again. Test your brakes by gently squeezing them, and then again by quickly squeezing them. The brake pads should be evenly spaced away from the rim and, when applied, should touch the wheel at the same time from both sides. The brake levers should react when squeezed, and you should not have to depress them completely. If your brakes pass this part of the test, check them again while on your bike, pedaling at a slow speed.

4. **Skewers:** You don't want these to be too loose or too tight. A good test is that you should be able to release your skewer with one hand, but not with one finger. After you have completed this test, the skewer should be properly tightened.

5. **Seat Post:** Tightness is also important here. If the bolt is not tight enough, your seat may work its way loose during the race, and basically make your bike unridable—unless you can stand for the entire second half of your Iron-distance bike leg! If you overtighten the bolt, you risk cracking certain types of frames. (I know of athletes who have done this the night before a race.) Get a good feel through practice of exactly how much your seat needs to be tightened, so you can avoid this mistake.

6. **Aero Bars:** If aero bars are not properly tightened, they can gradually loosen, especially if you are traveling on bumpy roads. This will cost you time and create a potentially dangerous situation. To test the tightness of your aero bars, stand in front of your bike, hold the end of your aero bars with both hands, and gradually apply more weight on them pressing down with your body weight. If you can move them, they are probably too loose. Tighten them too much, however, and you may strip the threads.

7. **Headset:** Having your headset bolt(s) tightened properly is one of the most important things you need to do. If this is loose, it can cause an accident. It needs to be snug, but not so tight that it damages your bike. Check with your bike mechanic on this one if you have any doubt about the proper tension.

8. **Helmet/Helmet Buckle:** Put your helmet on a couple of times and test your helmet buckle. The straps should be snug around your face, but not so tight that they restrict your breathing or head movement. If you cannot properly fasten your helmet buckle in the first transition, your race may be over. This creates a dangerous situation, and riding without a fastened helmet is a serious violation of USAT rules.

9. **Shoe Cleats:** Check your bike shoe cleats for cracks and excessive wear. Make sure they clip in and out of your pedals smoothly. Bring an extra set of cleats when traveling to races. Always make sure that the screws on the cleats are tight, as they may loosen while traveling.

10. **Tire-Changing Gear:** Don't just assume you have everything you need in your bike pouch. Take a quick inventory. For clincher tires I suggest two fresh tubes, three CO_2 cartridges and the proper adapter, and two of the plastic "tire irons." If you are not proficient at changing your tires, practice. This is something all cyclists should be able to do. To make practice fun, have a tire-changing competition with your cycling buddies or, for you brave souls, your spouse!

Bikes have been around for over a hundred years. While they have become more aerodynamic and sophisticated in certain ways, the basic mechanics are still pretty low-tech. Given this, it's somewhat surprising how much can go wrong. Far too often, races are ruined (or worse) due to mechanical problems. The best defense is to have your bike serviced frequently by a good mechanic and to invest the small amount of time necessary to ensure that your bike will perform safely and at its best. I hope this ten-point bike check helps to keep you fast and safe in your races.

• Cornering

Many beginning cyclists make turns by simply braking to slow down and then steering the bike through the turn. This is inefficient and can also be dangerous. You need to learn how to "carve" the turn quickly and safely.

As you approach a turn, you want to select an arc that will be both efficient and safe. You want to approach the turn wide, cut the apex in close, and then finish the turn wide again.

As you approach the turn you want to slide back in your saddle, increasing the weight on your rear wheel. As you enter the turn, your inside pedal should be up, with your knee extended out, and your outside pedal should be down. Keep your weight on the back of your seat and on the outside foot throughout the turn. Practice this technique at slow speeds and then gradually increase speed as you improve your cornering skills. Always be safe.

In wet conditions be more conservative. I don't recommend tilting the bike and leaning into the turn when the road surface is wet; this will often result in the dreaded "road rash." If it's a little wet, take speed off and cautiously make the turn with your bike in an upright position. And if it's very wet and slippery, I suggest you cycle indoors and save your cornering for another day.

Running Technique

Last but not least is running technique. You can definitely become faster and more efficient in this sport as well. In this section I will describe proper running technique and provide some tools to help you improve your form. I will also present special techniques for running on hills, as well as a few other running tips.

- **Upper Body**

Most importantly, run "tall." Your upper body greatly influences your lower body. The most common mistake I see among runners is leaning forward in the direction they are running. Stand up straight and erect. Hold your chin up and face straight ahead. Allow your shoulders to roll back slightly. Swing your arms forward and backward, not side to side. Relax your face, shoulders, and hands.

Years ago I learned of a great visualization trick to help perfect running form. It's called "Two Strings."

TAKE ACTION CHALLENGE: TWO STRINGS

Visualize one string coming out of the top of your head, pulling your head straight up toward the sky. This helps you to run "tall" and light on your feet, with your shoulders hanging loosely.

Visualize a second string coming out of the middle of your chest and pulling you forward in the direction you are running. This helps you to lead with your chest, and allows your shoulders to roll back slightly (sort of a chest-out, shoulders-back position).

In addition to improving your running form, this simple visualization exercise will also help you improve your breathing, lengthen your stride, and increase your overall efficiency. I have known about this trick for many years and still use it on almost every run. Please give it a try.

- **Lower Body**

Now for the lower body. With each stride, land on your heel, then roll forward onto the ball of your foot, and push off your toes. No side-to-side motion here either. Keep everything moving in a straight line, front to back.

Avoid bouncing or loping while you run. This is a common mistake. The energy you exert pushing up against gravity is wasted. You want to glide along close to the surface and only exert the minimal amount of energy necessary to resist gravity. To correct this technique flaw, try the following exercise.

TAKE ACTION CHALLENGE: BOUNCELESS RUNNING

While you are running, look at a stationary object off in the distance (50–100 meters). Possible objects include street signs, trees, and telephone poles. As you stare at the object, it should remain steady. If you find that it is bouncing in your view, begin reducing the upward push in your running gait, until the bouncing stops. To train yourself to always run smoothly, repeat this exercise several times on each run.

It is also useful to run on a treadmill in front of a mirror. The mirror provides continuous feedback on your form and helps you make needed adjustments.

- **Hill Running**

Hill running is challenging. As I said above regarding cycling technique, my recommendation is not to avoid hilly triathlons, but to meet the challenge head-on. Learn solid hill-climbing techniques and let the hills be someone else's problem, not yours.

I told you earlier that you should run "tall," facing straight ahead with your chin up. Well, there is one exception: hill running. When running up a hill, you need to lean forward slightly. I always tell my athletes to "lean into the hill." You also want to shorten your stride slightly and increase leg turnover slightly. You want to maintain your speed, but you will take shorter, quicker strides to do it.

TAKE ACTION CHALLENGE: TWENTY BREATHS

Hill running can be as difficult mentally as it is physically. Often runners stare at the top of the hill, yearning to get there. It's similar to the "watched pot never boils" syndrome: It seems to take forever.

Try the "Twenty Breaths" technique. Don't keep looking at the top of the hill and thinking about how far away it is. Instead look at the ground about 10 meters in front of you and count your breaths. After every twenty breaths, glance up and see how far away the top of the hill is. You will be able to see noticeable progress each time you look up, and this will make hill climbing psychologically easier.

To sum up, every training session is an opportunity to improve technique. Take full advantage of it. This is one of the best ways to improve race performance without increasing your training time. There is no reason to limit yourself with inefficient technique when, with no increase in training time, you can become faster.

CHAPTER 12

Mastering Transitions

"Pressure is nothing more than the
shadow of great opportunity."

—*Michael Johnson*

I find most Iron-distance triathletes overemphasize the urgency of transitions. They make the mistake of approaching the swim-to-bike transition in the Iron-distance much as they would in a sprint triathlon. They obsess over saving every possible second, sometimes to their detriment. I have seen athletes sprint out of the water with their hearts pounding, tripping over themselves to get their wetsuits off, then falling down, dropping equipment, and forgetting important items as they hastily change into their cycling gear. Then they literally jump onto their bike, knocking off bottles and energy gels, which will be sorely missed down the road.

Iron-distance transitions differ from short-course race transitions and should be approached differently. My comments in this chapter apply specifically to the Iron-distance.

In Iron-distance transitions, it's better to get it right than to get it fast. The transition is not the time to panic, it's the time for composure. We want to execute the transition efficiently, safely, and calmly; we want to go methodically from being a swimmer to being a cyclist. The risk of forgetting things and making other mistakes far outweighs the potential benefit of picking up 30 seconds. So don't be one of those athletes rushing through in a panic. Instead, practice your transition steps in training until you have them down to an almost robotic procedure.

Below I will tell you exactly how to execute a quick, simple, and effective transition for both T1 (the swim-to-bike transition) and T2 (the bike-to-run transition).

Swim-to-Bike Transition (T1) Plan

Race morning is not the time to plan your transition. It's best to have a plan well in advance and practice it weekly in training. This will not only help you to become more efficient, it will also greatly reduce your pre-race stress. Develop a sensible transition plan, practice it frequently, and stick to it.

Following is the type of swim-to-bike transition plan I have found to be most effective, along with some transition tips. Test this plan in your training and customize it to fit your needs and the specific details of your next race.

1. Run out of the water in a controlled and relaxed manner. As you head toward the equipment bag pickup area, unzip your wetsuit, pull your arms out of the sleeves, and pull your wetsuit down to your waist. Then remove your goggles and swim cap. Some races have volunteers available to help you strip off your wetsuit, right after you exit the water. This may be something you want to take advantage of, especially if you find that you find it difficult to remove your own wetsuit. While a small number of Iron-distance races do not permit wetsuits, most notably the Hawaii Ironman, the vast majority of them do.

2. Retrieve your cycling equipment bag in the designated area. **Tip:** Identify the position of your bag before the race, so you know exactly where to look for it in the crowded transition area.

3. Run with your equipment bag into the changing tent. Find an empty seat, put down your bag in front of the seat, finish removing your wetsuit (if you have not already removed it back at the water's edge with the assistance of one of the volunteers), and sit down. Then empty your cycling equipment bag onto the ground in front of you.

4. Put your socks on first. **Tip:** While some triathletes prefer not wearing socks, I recommend them as the possible time saving is far outweighed by the risk of getting a blister.

5. Put your cycling shoes on second. **Tip:** Some athletes prefer to attach their shoes to their pedals in advance. This is fine, but it's a

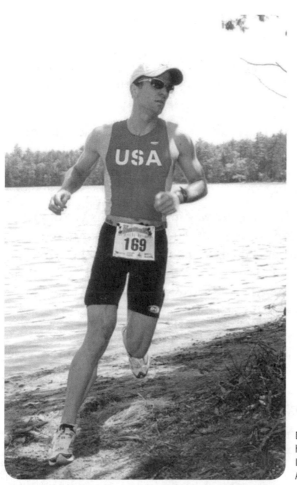

Dr. Scott Gac, married,
historian and author . . .
Iron-distance triathlete.
Photo Credit: Renee Shiller.

problem if you are planning to wear socks because they are likely
to become wet and soiled on your way to your bike.

6. Put on your singlet/top next. **Tip:** Many triathletes prefer wearing
   a one-piece tri suit, which can be worn right under your wetsuit
   and throughout the entire race.

7. Put your cycling glasses on. **Tip:** Some races allow you to attach
   these to your bike. This is somewhat risky, however, as they can
   be knocked off inadvertently by other triathletes or even race

volunteers, and either lost or damaged. So if you leave them on your bike, make sure they are secure.

8. Put your helmet on and buckle the chin strap. **Tip:** Don't ever forget this one. Besides being extremely important for safety reasons, it's usually an automatic DQ if you forget!

9. Put your wetsuit, swim cap, and goggles in the bag that held your cycling equipment and leave it with the race volunteer as you exit the changing tent. If a volunteer is available to assist you, they will often pack up your bag for you, but if not, it is your responsibility.

10. Run in a controlled and relaxed way to your bike. As you do, put sunscreen on any exposed areas of skin. **Tip:** Sometimes you can ask a helpful volunteer to do this for you in the changing tent while you attend to some of the previous steps. Wipe your hands off on your race suit after applying the sunscreen, as you don't want to have slippery hands on the bike.

11. Run cautiously with your bike to the bike-mounting line at the exit to the transition area. Once there, safely mount your bike and go! **Tip:** Prior to the race, do a practice walk-through from the changing tent to your bike, and from your bike to the transition exit, so that you don't waste any time searching for your bike or the exit on race day.

I recommend practicing these steps once a week during a Transition Workout session. Always practice these steps in the exact same order. The goal is to eliminate as much decision-making as possible. Ideally, you want to go through your planned steps efficiently and with machine-like accuracy.

Bike-to-Run Transition (T2) Plan

Most of my above comments hold true for the bike-to-run transition, although I notice a lot fewer athletes rushing through this one out of control—it's amazing what 7+ hours of racing will do to you. Just like the first transition, the bike-to-run transition requires a step-by-step routine, which we will practice every week until it becomes automatic. The goal is to execute the routine efficiently and without error after fatigue has set in.

Following is the step-by-step plan I use for the bike-to-run transition. Again, practice it and customize it to your needs and the particulars of your planned race.

1. Rack your bike (or hand it off to the appropriate race volunteer) and run in a relaxed and controlled way to the designated area to retrieve your equipment bag.

2. Take your bag and run to the changing tent. On the way, remove your cycling helmet.

3. When you arrive in the tent, find a seat, sit down, and empty your equipment bag in front of you.

4. Take off your cycling shoes and socks.

5. Put on your running socks and shoes. **Tip:** If your cycling socks are still dry, just keep them on for the run; if they are wet, it's best to put on a fresh, dry pair. Be prepared for either possibility.

6. Put on your running top. If required by the race, the race number should already be attached. Some races permit you to wear a race belt (note: race belts either have snaps to attach your number, or you use safety pins), in which case you can just pull your number around to your front. (Most races require your number to be worn in the front for running and in the back for cycling.) **Tip:** Wear a one-piece tri suit throughout the race to eliminate a couple of these clothes-changing steps.

7. Put your running hat on and either keep the same eyewear on or put on a clean pair.

8. Put sunscreen on as you exit the changing tent and grab a drink as you exit the transition area and begin the run course. Most races offer hydration at various points throughout the transition area, including at the start of the run course. **Tip:** Again, a helpful volunteer may be available to apply sunscreen as you attend to the other steps above.

As in the case of the swim-to-bike transition, practice your bike-to-run transition at least once a week. The transition session is usually the best place to do this, as it simulates race conditions.

AN IRONFIT MOMEMT

Excerpt from the Author's 2002 Hawaii Ironman Race Journal

I am wobbly from the rough swim as I run through the transition area to my bike. When I arrive I find no fewer than five volunteers there to assist me. Wow, this is service! I say "Thanks" to the one holding my helmet and I put it on. I say "Thanks" to the one holding my sunglasses and I put them on. I say "Thanks" to the one who had pulled my drinking straw out of my Jet Stream drinking system and was handing it to me. I take the straw and put it back into my Jet Stream. I say "Thanks" to the one who had taken one of my GU energy gels attached to my bike and hands it to me. I take it from him and reattach it to my bike. I say "Thanks" to the one holding my bike, as I take it from him. "Nice people!" I think as I ride away.

CHAPTER 13

Equipment Tips

"Everything from equipment to mental and
spiritual health can make the difference in
the outcome of a race."

—Mark Allen

will be honest: Triathlon equipment is complicated.

This is not like road racing, where you pretty much just need to show up with your running shoes on. There are so many types of equipment needed and there are so many competing products to choose from, all of them promising they are the best. It's difficult for most athletes to know what the best equipment choices are for them.

In this section, I explain the exact equipment requirements for your Iron-distance race and then provide tips on making intelligent choices in both training and racing equipment, as well as on how to avoid some potential pitfalls. First let's talk about what we need on race day.

Race Day Equipment

- **At the Swim Start**

When you enter the water, just before your Iron-distance race begins, you want to be wearing the following:

- Swim cap issued by the race (in some races these display your race number)

- Swim goggles

- Tri suit or swimsuit (underneath wetsuit)

- Wetsuit (if permitted by race)

- Sunblock

T1: The Swim-to-Bike Transition

After you exit the water, you will retrieve your T1 transition bag and take it to the changing tent. The following is what you should have in your T1 bag:

- Bike helmet (if not attaching to bike)

- Sunglasses (if not attaching to bike)

- Cycling shoes

- Cycling socks

- Race number (issued by race) attached to race belt or cycling top

- Cycling top (if not wearing tri suit)

- Sunblock

After leaving the changing tent you will retrieve your bike. Your bike should be set up with the following:

- Three bike bottles filled with energy drink

- Energy gels

- Tire-changing gear pack behind seat

- Two extra tubes (unless using tubular tires)

- Three CO_2 cartridges with appropriate adaptor

- Two plastic tire-changing levers

T2: The Bike-to-Run Transition

After dismounting your bike, you will retrieve your T2 gear bag. In this bag should be the following equipment:

- Running shoes

- Socks

- Running cap

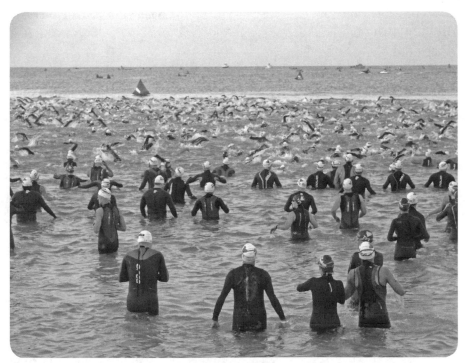

Photo Credit: Lynn Kellogg/www.trilifephotos.com.

- Energy gels

- Sunblock

• Special Needs Bags

Most Iron-distance races also provide "special needs bags," which can be retrieved around the midpoint of the bike course and the run course. Many athletes feel obligated to put something in these two bags, but this is one of those situations where less is more. If you don't have a special need, don't use them.

I have heard of athletes putting extra prescription medication and asthma inhalers in their special needs bags. This makes sense. But as far as extra food and items you can get at the aid stations anyway, I wouldn't bother. Given the time it takes to slow down (if not stop) in the middle of the race to retrieve these bags, it may not be worth it.

If possible, you want to bring everything you need with you on the bike; the only exception is replacement energy drink for after you finish your first three bottles.

Now that I have covered exactly what equipment we need during the race, following are my general tips on both training and racing equipment:

Running Equipment

• Training Shoes

Proper fit is important. Unless you already know the shoe and size that fits you best in a particular brand, you should go in person to buy. Find a good running store with personnel who have the experience to help you find the right fit for you.

Always have two pairs of running shoes and alternate them for each run; each pair will last longer than if you used it continuously. Keep track of the mileage on each pair. Shoes should be replaced after 55–70 hours (or about 500 miles).

Bring your used running shoes with you to the store when you purchase new ones. A good salesperson can learn things about your running mechanics from the wear pattern on the sole of the shoe and make better recommendations.

- **Racing Shoes**

Many triathletes use lightweight racing shoes, or racing flats, to shave off time in races. If you plan to use racing shoes, buy them at least two months before your race and use them once a week in training. Wearing new shoes for the first time in a race is a major rookie mistake. You need to break them in well in advance. New shoes may cause blisters, and that is not what you want during your Iron-distance marathon.

Do you need special racing flats for the Iron-distance? Possibly not—you may be better off with your training shoes. Running on the road produces an impact shock to your legs, which makes them increasingly sore the longer you are out there. Racing shoes sacrifice cushioning to save weight, so they do less than training shoes to pad the blows. It's a tradeoff: Eventually the soreness will slow you down more than the lightness will speed you up. I find that athletes who will be running the Ironman marathon over about 3:15 generally do better with training shoes instead of racing shoes.

It's difficult to keep your feet dry out on the course, and wet shoes cause blisters. Even if there is no rain, big puddles often form around the aid stations. Try to avoid these puddles as much as possible and, while it might be good on a hot day to pour some water over your head during the marathon, resist the temptation of drenching yourself to the point where water runs down your legs and collects in your shoes.

A good racing trick is to put Vaseline between your toes and on your heels and put on a fresh pair of socks before putting your racing shoes on. With practice you will be able to do this in 30 seconds, and the running comfort you gain will be well worth it.

AN *IRONFIT* MOMENT

Ryan Grote on Selecting Running Shoes (written in 2004)

Pro triathlete Ryan Grote is uniquely qualified on the topic of running shoes. Ryan has a passion for the Iron-distance, and in addition to being a former NCAA Track & Field All-American at 10,000 meters, he is now with The Running Company, a successful running specialty store with locations nationwide. In the following,

Ryan explains how to match an Iron-distance triathlete with the best shoe for them:

The purchase of running shoes is one of the most critical decisions you will make in selecting your arsenal of gear for Iron-distance racing. While considerably less expensive than buying a bike, running shoes are still quite technical and you need to be fit properly for the needs of your feet. This need not be a daunting and confusing process, as you can take some simple steps to inform yourself and find a knowledgeable running shoe specialist in your area. Go into the process with an open mind as to what kind of shoe you need, unless you are an experienced, competitive runner who has tended to stay with a brand or model of shoe without incident for a long period of time. If that is the case, the same rules should apply to your Iron-distance training and racing.

If you are new to the Iron-distance level of running, then try to find a running specialty store in your area, or ask other runners or running clubs in your area to recommend a store for your needs. It is good to be somewhat informed and knowledgeable about your shoes, but try not to put too much stock into magazine shoe reviews or catalog guidelines, as they are often just that: guidelines that are likely too general for your specific needs. For example, anybody could pick up a shoe review, read about any shoe in that review, and find qualities that sound sensible and attractive to them, but may not fit their needs. Shoes that are for very different types of feet or running gait can sound just right for you. A motion control shoe, intended for heavy over-pronators, those with usually flatter feet, will be described as supportive, sturdy, and durable. Who wouldn't want that? Probably about 90% of the population would not want or need that type of shoe. A neutral, cushioned shoe will be described as flexible, responsive, and cushioned. Again, who wouldn't want that? Well, the aforementioned over-pronator wouldn't want that type of shoe. That is not to say that the over-pronator does not want cushioning, but that type of foot strike needs more control, support, and guidance than others. All running shoes have cushioning, while some shoes have support features intended for different types of feet.

So, this is where it is helpful to find a running specialty store. Bring in the shoes you have been running in if you have some. This will help somebody to see from the wear on them what your tendencies are, or at the very least see what you've had and if they have worked well for you. There will likely be many shoes that could possibly work for you, and many that will not work for you. Try to use your past history and some ideas about your feet and running along with expert advice to come up with at least 3 different models of shoes to try on and walk or jog around in at the store. Be sure to try different brands, as each brand has a fit that will differ from another.

Again, try to avoid perceived notions about which brand or model is better for you initially. Just because a friend who has been successful at triathlon trains in a certain shoe does not mean it will work for you. You may find some brands to be too wide, or too narrow, or for the arch support to not feel comfortable to you. This is exactly why it is crucial for you to try on several different types after having some sound advice from an experienced runner.

Another thing to consider is price; you do not always need the most expensive shoe. Often the top-of-the-line, most expensive shoe in a line is heavier, as it contains all of the support and cushioning bells and whistles in their respective line. Many great runners and triathletes train successfully in shoes under $100. You do not always get more when you pay more. Usually the $80 retail price point will get you a shoe that features that company's respective cushioning technology through the whole shoe, which is important for the amount of running you will do for an Iron-distance triathlon. There is usually a big difference between a $60 shoe and an $80 shoe, but not a big difference between an $80 shoe and a $120 shoe in terms of their effectiveness for high mileage running. The lower end shoes will not have the cushioning and support features, and will break down more quickly. A good training shoe should last around 500 miles, a bit less for the lighter weight shoes or heavier weight athletes. Again, trying on different brands will allow you to decide which type of cushioning features are more comfortable; some brands are firmer, usually better for heavier runners, and some are lighter and softer.

Once you do have a new pair of shoes, break them in; do not take them right from the box to the roads. Walk around in them for a few hours or break them in lightly on a treadmill to make sure they are still comfortable. Your training will likely consist of more than 500 miles of running, so be prepared to buy more than one pair of shoes. If you will train and race in the same shoe, then make sure you buy your second pair of the shoes that have worked for you with enough time to put around 50 miles on them to break them in for the race. If you are racing more competitively and will use a racing flat or lighter trainer, then consider rotating different shoes while training. Most companies will offer lighter weight training shoes similar to their regular shoes. Often it makes sense to stick with the same brand as the shoes will have a similar fit and feel. If you will race in a lighter shoe, make sure you train in it at times, perhaps on your transition runs in brick workouts, as this will simulate how your legs and feet will feel in the Iron-distance race.

The process may seem complicated and vague, but it really is not. Do a little bit of research, but keep an open mind. Find a good running store, try on a number of different shoes and ask for a lot of help to find the right shoe for your feet. By the time you are running in your Iron-distance, your legs and feet will hurt enough, so you want to make sure that you are putting on a comfortable pair of shoes for the last 26.2 miles of your day.

Cycling Equipment

- **Triathlon Bike**

I am often asked which is better to have, a tri bike or a road bike. Either is fine.

Tri bikes position the rider in a slightly more aggressive way because the bike segment of the triathlon resembles a time trial. If all else is equal, I would recommend a tri bike. But if you are relatively new to the sport and you already have a good road bike, I would not rush out for a new tri bike; the road bike will do fine. I raced for many years on a standard road bike before getting my first tri bike.

What is the best tri bike? There is no right answer to this. There are many great tri bikes out there, and much has to do with personal preferences and body type. I find the Van Dessel All Systems Go to be the best tri bike for me, but I suggest you go to a couple of good bike shops and try out several models. Most shops only carry a few brands, so you may need to go to two or three shops to try a good sampling of the top bikes.

The most important element is fit. You can have the coolest looking bike out there, but if it's not fitted well for you, you are going to limit your speed potential and even risk injury. Have an experienced professional who understands triathlon positioning 1) help you to select the proper frame size, and 2) fit it properly to you. Don't leave this to a nice guy who has a summer job in the bike shop; it's just too important.

Learn all you can about your bike. It's great to have a top-notch bike mechanic to work on your bike, but he's not always going to be there. You should learn how to make at least minor adjustments and you should know how to give your bike a thorough bike safety check before every ride.

If you are going to fly to your race, you should also know how to pack your bike safely in a bike travel case, and you should know how to reassemble it safely when you arrive at your race.

Practice doing this in advance. Ask for help at the bike shop if you have problems.

AN IRONFIT MOMENT

Paul Levine on Bike Fitting (written in 2004)

Paul Levine, owner of Signature Cycles, located in New York City, Central Valley, NY, and Greenwich, CT, is on the leading edge of bike design and bike fitting technology. Paul is also the program director and an instructor at Serotta's Institute of Professional Bike Fitting, one of the premier bike fitting training facilities in the world. In the following, Paul provides guidance on how an Iron-distance triathlete can find the optimal bike fit:

The optimal long course triathlon position is not necessarily the best aerodynamic position, but it's the one that finds the best balance between comfort, power, efficiency, and aerodynamics.

Airflow characteristics over the body change at 18 miles per hour, and again at 29 miles per hour. Your bike fit should reflect the speeds with which you will travel. A long course triathlete should not be as concerned with aerodynamics as a Time Trial cyclist. Typically the TT rider needs only to stay in his position for less than one hour while he maintains speeds approaching 29 MPH. The goal of the long course triathlete is to stay aero as long as possible without creating a high metabolic cost to maintain their aero position. It is the athlete who can "whisper the loudest" on the bike who will be the most ready to run the marathon without excessive muscular fatigue or biomechanical stress.

When preparing a bicycle for a long course event, it is important to set the bike up for maximum efficiency. An efficient position is one that allows for a maximizing of the ratio of power to drag, while maintaining proper biomechanics to allow one to pedal properly and sit comfortably on the bike. It is quite common to be too aero, thus not allowing one to produce sufficient power or to ride comfortably. There are four key elements to achieving a good efficient long course triathlon position:

1. **A flat torso:** A flat torso makes the biggest impact on reducing drag on the bike. We create the flat torso by using aero bars. The use of aero bars gets the torso out of the way of the wind and properly set up will allow the skeletal structure of the upper arms to support the weight of the athlete, rather than loading the muscular system.

2. **A forward seat angle:** A tri position uses a more forward seat position than a road bike, allowing the femur/torso angle to open up, while maintaining the low-profile position needed. It is important not to have too forward a position, as this will lead to loss in power, poor pedal mechanics, along with overall poor balance on the bicycle.

3. **Narrow flat arms:** The athlete's arms should be as flat as possible without causing discomfort in the trapezoids, wrists, and forearm

contact points. The arm width should shadow the athlete's thighs, and in fact, being too narrow can increase drag.

4. **Adaptation:** In order for one to be efficient on a triathlon bike the athlete needs to ride it at least once a week. The athlete needs to adapt to producing power, pedaling efficiently, consuming and digesting nutrients, and becoming completely comfortable in their event specific position.

The basic positioning process for a long course triathlete follows the same basic fitting rules as fitting of any other bicycle. For an athlete to cycle efficiently in a long course event the athlete must be positioned in such a way that their power output is not compromised, which means staying within the flexibility limits of the athlete. An athlete's range of motion must be accessed for their hamstrings, hip flexors, hip rotators, and spine prior to determining their most efficient long course position. An athlete should never be positioned to be in their end range of motion for any of their muscles or tendons about their joints.

The fitting of the athlete begins by positioning the saddle height and set back. Triathlon saddles need to be lower than road bike saddles to accommodate the increased pelvic tilt, which raises the hip sockets, increasing the reach to the pedals. The starting position of the saddle height should be 3 to 5 mm lower than the athlete's road bike saddle. The angle at the knee when the foot is at the bottom of the pedal stroke should be approximately 145 degrees.

A good starting point for saddle setback is to cut the setback of the saddle in half from the athlete's road bike. A knee-over-pedal spindle measurement should be taken from the tibial plateau (the bump on the outside of the front of the knee) and should be approximately +/- 1 cm.

Once the saddle is roughly positioned the front of the bicycle can now be addressed. The amount of drop an athlete can run from the saddle to the handlebars will vary significantly from athlete to athlete depending on their individual flexibility. A rule of thumb is you can lower an athlete until the point at which the athlete begins to hyperflex their spine and/or hyperextend their neck.

The reach of the handlebars is significant and is the one area that is most mispositioned. The idea is that the shoulder socket should be roughly 1 to 2 cm behind the elbow joint. This allows for the skeletal structure of the upper arm to support the weight of the athlete having the least metabolic cost for creating structural stability. Many short torso athletes need to modify their position from these guidelines whereas their knees may hit the backs of their upper arms.

By applying the above basic rules of bike set-up you will typically increase the performance of most athletes. The essential elements of comfort, power, and efficiency must be addressed along with aerodynamics. Strictly focusing on aerodynamics will result in slower bike times. The goal is to be comfortable and stay in the aero position. All the work you do to get an aero position doesn't do any good if you are not in it.

• Bike Tires and Tubes

I am always surprised at how many triathletes don't know how to change a tire, don't have the right equipment to do it, or cannot do it efficiently in race conditions. Wishing you won't get a flat is not a good strategy. Eventually it happens to everyone.

The ability to change a tire quickly is especially important in Iron-distance racing, where you have time to overcome this setback. In a sprint race, a flat tire is usually a disaster. In Iron-distance racing, if you can change your tire in less than 4 minutes it probably won't even cost you a place in your age group, let alone stop you from successfully finishing the race. I recommend that you carry two extra tubes, two plastic tire-changing levers, and three CO_2 cartridges, for those with clincher tires. Make sure the equipment in your changing kit is in good repair.

Make it your goal to change a flat tire at least once a month. If you are lucky enough not to have any flats in a particular month, change one anyway on the last day of the month, just to stay sharp and in practice.

When you are resting in your hotel room in the days leading up to your Iron-distance race, practice changing a tire with a stopwatch once a day, and try to compete against your own personal record. This simulates changing a tire under the pressure of the clock. My wife and I sometimes have a friendly competition with this. After a "ready-set-go," we race each other to see who can change the tire fastest. This is a great confidence builder going into the race.

In the 2000 Ironman New Zealand I suffered two flat tubes on those rough country roads. Thanks to practice and being prepared with the right tire-changing gear, I was able to get back on the road quickly. I didn't set a personal best that day, but I was able to battle back to second master overall and win a slot for Hawaii. Not such a bad day after all!

• Cycling Shoes

I suggest buying a high-quality pair of cycling shoes well before the race date and spending several months breaking them in. You never want to break in new equipment just before the race.

Cycling shoes should be snug but comfortable. You need to have them on for several hours. Try them on with the same type of socks you plan to wear in the race and then continue to train with that same type of socks, especially on your long rides, which best simulate race conditions.

Some experienced triathletes start the bike segment of the race with their shoes already attached to their pedals. They put their feet into them while they are in motion. I don't recommend this for most Iron-distance triathletes. It's too risky and the time savings are minimal. The transition is crowded, you may be a little disoriented from the swim, and collisions with other riders are possible. Take a couple of extra seconds and get your shoes on correctly and safely. It's a long race. The value of a couple seconds here is far outweighed by the risk of a major setback early in the race.

• Bike Helmet

Find a high-quality, protective, aerodynamic helmet that is snug yet comfortable. You should not be able to slide the helmet easily around on your head once the chin strap is fastened.

Always tightly fasten your chin strap before mounting your bike, and don't unfasten it until you have handed off your bike to the volunteers and you are on your way to the run transition tent. To do so is against the rules and just plain stupid. This is not an area to cut corners. Even the best cyclists come in unwelcome contact with the road from time to time.

Swim Equipment

- **Wetsuit**

The fit is key. You want a suit that is comfortable and allows for easy breathing and a good range of arm motion, but the suit must also fit snugly and produce little drag. Don't buy this item from a catalog or over the Internet. Go to a good tri shop and try on several types and sizes until you find the one that fits you best.

Wear your wetsuit in training at least once or twice a month. You want to become comfortable with it. Don't wait until race morning to put on your wetsuit for the first time in several months.

In this area you can buy speed. Many of the top manufacturers offer more flotation and greater range of motion in their top-of-the-line wetsuit. Within a certain brand, the $550 wetsuit is usually going to be faster than the $350 suit. The full wetsuit, with long sleeves and legs, is usually faster than the sleeveless suit or the short suit.

- **Tri Suit**

I prefer a one-piece tri suit to a swimsuit. You can wear them throughout the entire race, so you don't lose time changing clothes. They are usually made to be aerodynamic and cool. Some even have a pocket in the back, which is great for carrying energy gels.

- **Swim Goggles**

Try on many different pairs to find the style that fits you best. This is difficult for many, but you really need to find a style that is comfortable and provides an airtight fit. To test this, press the goggles over your eyes. They should stay on your face, even without the strap on your head.

I recommend that you buy two pairs of goggles and rotate them in training. Then, bring them both on race morning. If you want to see panic, watch somebody break a goggle strap 60 seconds before the start of an Ironman race. Be prepared and have a backup.

The shaded type is often recommended for swimming outdoors. Try these out to make sure you like them before using them in a race. I find they make it hard to see during early morning swims when the sun isn't quite up yet (and I find they don't offer much help anyway if the swim course forces you to look into the sun). I use the non-shaded indoor goggles for early morning swim starts.

- **Swim Cap**

The race organizers usually supply an official swim cap for the race, but bring one along for training in the days leading up to the race.

Even if your hair is very short, train with a cap at least some of the time so you will feel comfortable wearing one on race day. Also practice swimming with your goggles under (not over) your swim cap. The cap helps you keep from losing them during crowded open-water swim starts.

Always wear a brightly colored swim cap when swimming in open water (and always swim with a partner).

Other Equipment

- **Heart Rate Monitor**

As you know from the chapter on heart rate training (Chapter 6), this one is essential. If you are serious about time-efficient training, you need to have a heart rate monitor. They are lightweight and most find them to be relatively comfortable.

There are many different models to choose from. The most popular type includes a chest strap and wristband receiver which provides a continuous heart rate reading of beats per minute. There are many styles and features available. Personally, I am not that interested in all of the bells and whistles. Simple and reliable is better. All you need is a basic model with a continuous heart rate readout. Heart rate monitors are available at bike shops, running stores, fitness centers, and through triathlon equipment catalogs and Web sites.

• Sun Protection

This one is easy to overlook, yet it is literally a matter of life and death. Training and racing in the hot sun is dangerous. There are over 1 million Americans with skin cancer and the number is growing at record rates. If you are an active person who spends a lot of time outdoors, you are in the highest risk group; if you are fair-skinned, you are in the highest end of the highest risk group.

Use sunblock when training outdoors. When it comes to racing, don't rely solely on the race volunteers to provide you with sunblock; bring your own. I recommend including sunblock with your other gear at both transitions. I suggest that you use it liberally before the swim, and again during each transition.

CHAPTER 14

Race and Pre-Race Strategies

"When you go for it 100%, when you don't
have that fear of 'what if I fail,' that's when
you learn. That's when you are really living."

—*Mark Allen*

It is amazing how many people spend up to a year of their lives training and sacrificing for their Iron-distance goal, and then just show up at the race without a plan. You can easily identify these athletes on race mornings. They are the ones with the "deer in the headlights" look. Both a race plan and a pre-race plan are crucial for Iron-distance success.

How many days before the race should you arrive? What should you eat in the last few days before the race? How much sleep should you get? How much training should you do in the final days? Where should you position yourself on the starting line?

These are all decisions that should be made well in advance of arriving at the race location. With all of the pre-race anxiety that is sure to arise, an athlete needs to have a clear pre-race and race plan.

In this section I explain the importance of both a race plan and a pre-race plan and discuss the key elements of the race that a successful race plan will address: race fueling, course segmentation, heart rate, and exactly what you should do in the final days leading up to the race. I also present a strategy for those whose goal is only to finish within the 17-hour time limit.

Race Fueling Strategy

One of the most underestimated elements of successful Iron-distance racing is race day fueling. For various reasons, many triathletes arrive at an

Iron-distance starting line having spent far too little time thinking about what and when they will eat and drink, and making the necessary preparations. Many of them learn that the difference between a good fueling plan and a poor fueling plan can be measured in hours.

Why is this racing element often taken too lightly? Some athletes feel that they should "eat how they feel." They believe that when their body needs something, it will let them know. Other athletes simply carry over their fueling plans from short-course racing. Whatever they normally do for shorter competitions, they do for the Iron-distance. Still other athletes hope they can simply copy the eating plan of a successful triathlete. Maybe they read something about what one of the top triathletes eats and drinks, and they decide to give it a try on race day.

Let's start out by addressing these approaches. At first glance, "Eat how you feel" seems sensible. The problem is that there is a significant lag between what you need and how you feel: By the time you feel thirsty, you may already be dehydrated. If you eat and drink how you feel, you may very well get behind in both hydration and calories—and have one of the longest days of your life out there!

How about using your short-course fueling plan? You might get lucky, but in most cases what you need to get through a 1- to 3-hour race is very different from what you need for a 9- to 17-hour race.

As for copying another athlete's fueling plan, without testing the plan in race-like conditions, it's a shot in the dark. What works for one person doesn't always work for another. If it did, race fueling would be a snap.

The best strategy is to test and perfect your fueling plan well before your race. The Iron-distance athletes I coach generally use their Long Bike and Long Run days for this purpose. These are the best occasions for trying out fueling options because they simulate race conditions most accurately.

In these sessions we stick to a specific fueling plan, and then we examine the results and make changes as necessary. We then test the revised plan in the next training opportunity. We usually start this process at least 10 weeks before the actual race.

Through working with many athletes, I have found that the average-sized male athlete (say about 160 pounds) can usually benefit from a plan that includes about 1,000 calories on the morning of the race, followed by about 500 calories per hour, consumed evenly during the race. And for the average-sized female athlete (say about 130 pounds) usually the best plan includes about 800 calories the morning of the race, followed by about 400 calories per hour, consumed evenly during the race.

Every athlete is a little different, and body size and food preferences need to be considered. However, if an athlete consumes less than his or her calories per hour, he or she will often run out of energy ("bonk") in the mid to late stages of the race. If he consumes more than his or her calories per hour, he or she will often feel too full and possibly experience stomach upset.

The following is a plan that has worked successfully for many average-sized athletes I have worked with. Make modifications based on your size and food choices, and most importantly, test it several times in training before trying it in a race.

- **Pre-Race Fueling**

  1. Upon waking (3 hours before the race), eat three of your favorite energy bars. Any good bar will do, as long as it is balanced in proteins, fats, and carbohydrates. They should also be bars that you have found to be easy to digest, which is just what you want when you have the pre-race jitters. Total calories: 600.

  2. Between "breakfast" and race time, gradually drink two bike bottles of your favorite energy drink. Total calories: about 300.

  3. About 10 to 15 minutes before the start, just before you enter the water for your warm-up, consume one GU energy gel. I find that this pre-start GU gel, in addition to topping off my calories, gives me a burst of energy just when I need it. Total calories: 100. Total calories for steps 1 through 3: about 1,000.

- **Fueling on the Bike**

  1. Upon mounting your bike and settling in, consume one GU gel. Set your watch and for the remainder of the bike consume another GU every 25 minutes.

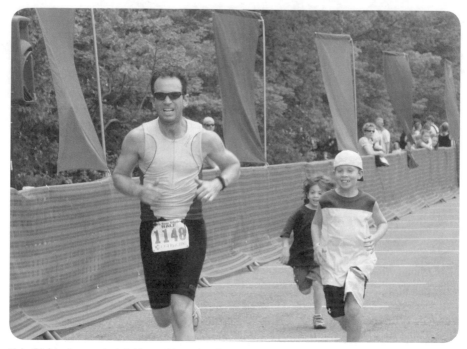

Eric Siskind, married, father of two, business executive . . . Iron-distance triathlete.
Photo Credit: Wendy Siskind.

2. Begin consuming energy drink. Finish a bottle every 35 to 40 minutes. Steps 4 and 5 combined will work out to an average of about 500 calories per hour.

- **Fueling on the Run**

  1. Continue consuming a GU gel every 25 minutes during the run, and sufficient energy drink at every aid station to maintain the 500-calorie-per-hour target. Some athletes like to switch over to cola on the run; however, it is important to test cola in your training, because not everybody tolerates it well. Whether you decide to stay with energy drink or switch to cola on the run, you should estimate in advance the quantity of beverage you need to consume at each aid station to maintain your 500-calorie target.

While the plan above has worked well for many, again it is important that you test your plan several times in training before using it in an actual race. As you test your plan, make modifications as necessary to find the exact plan that energizes you the best.

Aid Station Tips:

> *"It's a long race, but it's catered."*
> —Ironman Champion Paul Huddle

The following are some tips to consider as you put your fueling plan together:

- Find out what replacement drink the race will be serving and practice with it for several weeks prior to the race.

- Keep your plan simple. Choose food that is easy to carry. The simpler your plan, the more likely it is that you will be able to follow it.

- Try not to rely completely on outside assistance for your fuel. Bring your own food with you if possible. In the above example, this was energy gels, however, some athletes prefer various types of energy bars. This way you can avoid having to stop or slow down as often, and you won't be derailed by handoff errors or shortages.

- Consume your calories as evenly as possible. Set your watch and consume your calories and hydration evenly over each hour of the entire race. Don't put yourself in a position of having to play catch-up.

- Stick with your plan. Every race has its ups and downs. Don't let the rough patches knock you off your plan. Hang in there and stick with your well-tested plan.

- Check the race Web site, or ask the race director about where the aid stations are positioned on the course and what they will be serving.

The bike aid stations are usually about 10 miles apart and the run stations are about 1 mile apart. This is important to know so you can accurately plan the timing of your fueling strategy.

- Drink choices typically include water and energy drink on the bike, and these same two plus defizzed cola on the run. Food choices include energy gels, energy bars, bananas, and sometimes even cookies and soup for those still racing after dark. Find out exactly what will be served and practice several weeks in advance with any foods and drinks you plan to use. Race day is not the time for experimentation.

Course Segmentation Strategy

One of the best techniques for making the 140 miles of the Iron-distance race seem more manageable and less intimidating is to segment the course in your mind before the race.

Mentally break the course into smaller, more digestible pieces. Then on race day, instead of visualizing the enormity of the entire course, just focus on the section you are currently on. This is so much easier on your mind and attitude.

When you complete one section, just put it behind you, and mentally move onto the next section. Focus on completing the segment you are currently in. Do not dwell on getting to the finish line, which may be 100 miles and several hours away.

For example, I break the Hawaii Ironman bike course up in my mind into eight segments, which range in length from 7 miles to 20 miles. When I am on one particular segment, I try to focus only on completing that segment, and I don't allow myself to think about any other segments. Try it. It works.

When you drive the course before the race, pick out landmarks and organize the race into sections in your mind. Learn the approximate distance of each section, and think about how long it will take you to get through each one. For example, here is my detailed segmentation of the Hawaii Ironman bike course:

1. From the bike start, complete the loop through town and then head out on the Queen K Highway to the airport (about 15 miles).

2. From the airport, continue on the Queen K to the entrance of Waikoloa (about 15 miles).

3. From the Waikoloa entrance to the turnoff onto the Queen K onto Rt. 290 (about 10 miles).

4. From Rt. 290 to the turnaround point in Hawi (about 20 miles).

5. Back from Hawi to the turnoff onto the Queen K (about 20 miles).

6. Pass the Waikoloa entrance on the Queen K (about 10 miles).

7. Pass the airport on the Queen K (about 15 miles).

8. To the bike-to-run transition (about 7 miles).

Thus, eight manageable segments totaling 112 miles. Try this same technique for any Iron-distance bike course. And don't forget, you also want to segment the swim and run courses.

Heart Rate and Pacing Strategy

After mistakes in fueling, the next most common mistake in Iron-distance racing is to race at too high a heart rate. Like under-fueling or under-hydrating, an elevated heart rate will lead to the dreaded "bonk" in the mid to late stages of the race.

The best way to maximize your performance is to complete the entire race in your aerobic heart rate range. I repeat: The best way to pace yourself through your Ironman is to stay 100% aerobic. No higher than Z2 all the way.

Allow your heart rate to select your pace, not the other way around. Maintain a comfortable, aerobic heart rate as much as you possibly can. As we saw in Chapter 6, the aerobic system powers us with an almost endless fuel supply: fat and oxygen. When your heart rate rises above your aerobic range, the fuel mix shifts and you begin to burn the short-term energy sources required by the anaerobic system. These short-term energy sources will be depleted long before an Iron-distance triathlon is over, and running them down will have residual effects that will hurt your overall performance.

The best advice is to keep it as aerobic as possible. Stay in your Z2 range. If running up a hill starts to force your heart rate up out of your aerobic range, back off just a bit, regain your composure, and settle back into your aerobic zone as quickly as possible.

Wear your heart rate monitor in the race if you feel you need it to keep you in the proper zone. Mark Allen, one of the greatest Ironmen ever, raced with a heart rate monitor, so you will be in very good company.

The "I Just Want to Finish under 17 Hours" Strategy

This section is not for everybody. It is written for the athlete who perhaps only has time for the "Just Finish" training program in Chapter 7. For this athlete victory is defined as completing the Iron-distance before the cutoff time of 17 hours. In a way these are the smart ones, as they get a lot more for their entrance fees than the athletes finishing under 10 hours.

In addition to the overall cutoff time of 17 hours, there are interim cutoff times for each individual sport. An athlete must make these interim hurdles to be allowed to continue. It is important to build these specific time limits into your plan if your goal is a sub-17-hour finish.

In the following points, I present my tips on how you can best work within the interim cutoff times to put together your plan to make it to the finish line by midnight.

- ### Just Finish Swim Strategy

The swim section is crucial. Make sure well ahead of race time that you can make it in under the swim cutoff of 2 hours and 20 minutes.

You have 140 minutes to swim 3,800 meters. That's about 3 minutes and 40 seconds for each 100 meters (38 of them!). Practice this pace in training, so you can be sure that you are ready. Open water swimming is typically slower than pool swimming, so also allow for some cushion.

A great way to do it is to swim at a slightly faster pace and then take short rests at predetermined times. For example, take a 1-minute rest after every 15 minutes of swimming. Here one of the great benefits of a wetsuit is that it allows you to just stop and rest in the water, without having to exert much energy to stay afloat.

Note: Some Iron-distance races have slightly different time limits, but most are 2:20. Check with the race you are planning to enter.

- **Just Finish Bike Strategy**

The bike cutoff time is usually 10.5 hours after the start of the race. Therefore, if you need all of the 2:20 on the swim segment, and say a comfortable 10 minutes for the transition, you will have about 8 hours to complete the bike segment. This works out to an average pace of about 14 miles per hour.

Try this pace during your Long Rides in training to be sure that you are ready for it. As with the swim, you may want to consider a slightly faster pace and plan for some brief breaks for resting, fueling, and using the bathroom. One approach would be to stop for a planned 5-minute break at an aid station after every 2 hours of cycling.

- **Just Finish Run Strategy**

Let's say you used all of your allowable time on the swim (2:20), you had a 10-minute transition, and then you used all of the remaining allowable time on the bike (8:00). You are within all of the interim time limits, and you are left with 6.5 hours to complete the marathon.

This works out to an average marathon pace of just under 15 minutes per mile. While this pace is probably not quite "walkable" after this long day (unless you are a really good walker), it is a pace that can be accomplished with a well-planned "walk-jog" approach.

If you think you may find yourself in this situation, I suggest the following strategy: Walk 5 minutes, jog 10 minutes, walk 5 minutes, jog 10 minutes, etc. Practice this approach in training to get a feel for it. If you can average about 20 minutes per mile on your walk and about 12 minutes per mile on your jog . . . you will achieve your Iron Dream!

- **Other Just Finish Tips**

Just Finish athletes will spend much more time out on the course than their swifter competitors, and that exposure intensifies the challenge. Here are a few more tips:

- Keep up with your fueling and hydrating. You may find that you are not exactly enjoying the cuisine after a while, but it is important to stay focused and stick to your fueling and hydrating plan.

- Wear well-tested, comfortable running shoes and socks, and keep your feet dry. While it may be helpful to pour cool water on your head on a hot day, try to keep your feet as dry as possible. Wet running shoes can lead to blisters, which believe me, you don't want.

- Attitude is crucial. Stay positive. Smile to the spectators. Thank the volunteers. Keep reminding yourself that this is your day, and that you are in the process of achieving something truly spectacular.

Pre-Race Strategy: The Countdown

The final few days before your Iron-distance race can be a stressful time. You have worked so long and hard, and you have made such an enormous personal investment in this one day. It's totally natural to feel nervous.

However, instead of taking steps to make the best of these last days and to reduce pre-race stress, many athletes actually complicate it. Some athletes make the mistake of putting off tasks and decisions until these last few days, greatly increasing their stress level. Instead of relaxing and preparing themselves mentally for the race, they are running around town trying to take care of last-minute details.

Some athletes spend a lot of time over the last couple of days at the race expo. They are on their feet and often in the hot sun for hours. Both of these things should be avoided, as they will leave you tired and dehydrated. I have even seen athletes get sunburned in the days before the race, which of course is going to hurt their performance.

This is something I would refer to as a "rookie mistake." You are so excited about being at your first Iron-distance that you want to hang out at the expo and take in the experience. I can certainly understand this, but I would suggest that you arrive a few days early if you want to cruise the expo. Save the last couple of days to rest, gather your strength, and prepare mentally for your race.

Other athletes are so nervous that they don't know what to do with themselves. They fill the void with training. Ouch! Another rookie mistake. As you can see in the IronFit training programs in Chapter 7, our training should be very light in that last week. We want to be making deposits in our energy bank, not drawing on it.

Plan for plenty of rest in the final couple of days. Get your feet up as much as possible. Stay out of the sun. Bring a good book or a CD and find your calm.

The best way to head off any of these pre-race mistakes is to write out a 3-day pre-race plan. I call this approach "The Countdown" because it starts 3 days before the race and then counts down the planned events until the time of the actual race. It includes meals, sleep, training, registering for the race, equipment, bike drop-off, etc. By preparing this plan and not having to make constant decisions on what to do and when to do it, you can be relaxed and confident going into your race.

I have successfully utilized this technique with many of the athletes I have worked with. It may sound like nothing more than a simple to-do list, but it's actually a powerful tool that can help you begin the race physically rested and mentally focused for a breakthrough. To help you visualize what this looks like, here is a sample Countdown:

Sample Countdown

- **Thursday**

6:00 a.m.	Awake, eat, drink, and dress
7:30	Easy 30-minute swim, easy stretching
8:30	Rest period (read, listen to music, watch television, etc.)
10:30	Register for race
11:30	Early lunch
1:00 p.m.	Rest period
5:00	Race meeting
6:00	Race pasta dinner
7:30	Rest period
9:00	Bedtime

- **Friday**

6:00 a.m.	Awake, eat, drink, and dress
8:00	Easy 20-minute run, easy stretch
9:00	Organize race gear, safety check bike

10:00	Snack and hydration
10:15	Rest period
2:00 p.m.	Eat early "dinner"
3:30	Check in bike and gear bags at transition area; practice walk-through
5:00	Organize remaining gear and food for race morning
5:30	Rest period; snack and hydration
9:00	Bedtime

- **Saturday**

4:00 a.m.	Awake, eat, drink, and dress
4:45	Leave for race check-in
5:00	Check in and body markings
5:20	Check bike, review transition area, and use bathroom
6:30	Good luck kiss!
6:40	Enter water for warm-up (See warm-up tips on next page)
6:50	Find predetermined position on starting line (See starting line tips on next page)
7:00	Race start!

Note how much rest time is built into the Countdown, and how much of a time cushion is included with each activity. Now it's your turn. The following exercise challenges you to plan your own Countdown.

TAKE ACTION CHALLENGE:
THE COUNTDOWN

Write your own 3-day Countdown. Check the specific details of your Iron-distance race. What time is registration? Gear check-in? Bike check-in? The pre-race meeting? The time the transition area opens on race day? And all other relevant details.

After you have gathered this key information, build a sensible Countdown plan around it. Include plenty of time for rest periods. Allow a comfortable time margin for each activity. This is your opportunity to ensure everything is taken care of. A good Countdown will greatly reduce your stress and free you to just relax, put your feet up, and prepare yourself mentally to enjoy one of the experiences of a lifetime.

STARTING LINE STRATEGY AND PRE-RACE WARM UP

The most common type of Iron-distance race start is an in-water start. It is usually set up in the water 30 to 50 meters from the beach and is marked by buoys. The competitors must line up behind the line created by these buoys.

You should line up at the start according to your swim ability and experience: faster swimmers in front, slower swimmers in the back. These starts can be crowded and some bumping often occurs, so it is safest to seed yourself properly.

The swim courses are usually either rectangular or triangular in shape. In addition to your relative swimming speed, let the direction of the first turn also help you to determine your optimal position at the start. If the first turn is to the right, the fastest swimmers will not only line up in the front, they will also line up to the right side of the front, so they can achieve the shortest line to the first turn. This is helpful to know, because if you are a slower swimmer or somewhat on the timid side, you may then want to select a position to the left side. You will be giving up very little in distance, and probably assuring yourself of a less crowded and less stressful swim. If you are really concerned about swimming in a crowd, and would prefer completely open water, just wait for 30 to 60 seconds to start after the gun goes off. Giving up this time is meaningless in a 140-mile race, but the peace of mind will be well worth it. After all, why stress over it? We want it to be a fun and safe experience.

These same tips apply to the other common type of race start, the beach start. With beach starts there is typically a starting line just like a running race. When the starting gun sounds, the athletes run down to the water (usually 30 meters or less), enter the water, and begin to swim. As with in-water starts, consider both your relative swim speed and the direction of the first turn, in selecting your starting position.

With either in-water starts or beach starts, you should enter the water at least 20 minutes before the start for a light warm-up. I suggest starting your warm-up with 3 to 5 minutes of easy relaxed swimming. Then 3 to 5 minutes of 30 second pick-ups (slight increases in pace), each followed by 30 seconds of easy swimming. Finally, 3 to 5 more minutes of easy relaxed swimming. Claim your selected position on the starting line, at least 5 to 10 minutes before the start. The closer you want to be to the front line, the earlier you should arrive within this 5 to 10 minute time range. **Tip:** *Waiting for the start can be stressful. Stay positive while you wait. Smile and wish your fellow athletes a good race. You will feel better, and so will they.*

CHAPTER 15

Mental Training

"Life has less to do with what happens to
you than it does with how you deal with
what happens to you."

—*Anonymous*

Control your thoughts. It's the most important mental skill you can
develop for success in endurance racing. It sounds so simple, but for
most it is not.

It's easy to be positive and confident when things are going smoothly,
but it's another story when things aren't so good. It's easy to become negative and let self-doubts and fears take hold of your thoughts. Successfully
dealing with this is as important as any other aspect of endurance racing.

What you think about during the race, how you deal with your fears, and
how you react to events is crucial to your success. It is not so important what
happens to you. What is truly important is how you deal with what happens
to you.

Ronald Reagan, one of the most famous optimists, liked to tell a story
about a boy who walked into the barn and stepped into a pile of manure. A
wide smile came across the boy's face and he said, "I know there must be a
pony in here somewhere." This type of optimism made Ronald Reagan a success at virtually everything he attempted in his life. Ask yourself right now:
If you walked into a barn and stepped in manure, what would be your first
words? I suspect they would not be words you would want to say in front of
your children!

To make an understatement, Iron-distance racing is difficult. As Mark
Allen once said, the Ironman "reduces you to the most basic element of
yourself." You will have unbelievably difficult times out there, times when

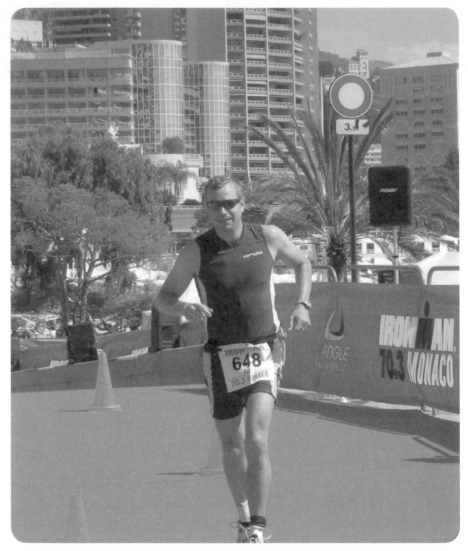

Paul Le Houillier, married, father of two, business executive . . . Iron-distance triathlete. *Photo Credit: Brigitt Heger.*

you fear you will not be able to make it and everything you worked for will be a loss. We need to prepare mentally for moments like these. We need to train our minds and condition our thought patterns to react in the right way to these mental challenges.

Many start out saying, "I'm a tough guy and I will handle it." But the truth is you really don't know until you are in that situation. Many an Iron-distance veteran has been reduced to tears by this race. You must anticipate these rough patches and prepare for them. The key is to train your mind, just as you train your body, to deal with the doubts and fears that are certain to come.

In the next section I will take a closer look at fears and self-doubts and then present my favorite mental training techniques for controlling your thoughts.

Fears and Self-Doubts

Mark Twain once wrote, "Courage is resistance to fear, mastery of fear—not absence of fear." This quote is one of my favorites, because it captures the essence of what courage is and how it can make an individual a success in endurance racing and in life in general. Courage does not mean you are without fear. Courage means you have fear but you have learned to deal with it in a positive way.

There is no shortage of fear and self-doubt in most athletes when they step up to the starting line of an Iron-distance race. What we need to do is to understand our fears, to put them into perspective, and to use them as powerful motivators for success.

Fear can be the biggest obstacle to achieving our goals. To a large extent, we are all controlled by our fears. The choices we make every day are partially driven by the various fears we have accumulated throughout our lives.

When you break it down to its most basic components, there are only two basic fears: the fear of death or injury, and the fear of embarrassment. And while avoiding death or injury seems like a pretty good idea, developing irrational fears related to death will limit our lives and reduce our freedoms.

As for embarrassment, what can I say? This falls into the category of, "You don't regret the things you did in life; you regret the things you didn't do." Please get over this one. If you are not doing something for fear of embarrassment, you can bet someday you will regret your inaction.

Many fears are irrational. For the average American the odds of being attacked by a shark are about 1 in 7 million, yet countless numbers of people have denied themselves the enjoyment of the ocean at any depth deeper than their ankles since they first saw *Jaws* four decades ago. Likewise, the odds of dying in a commercial airline crash for the average American are about 1 in 1 million, yet thousands of people avoid seeing the world for fear of air travel.

These are irrational fears. Compared to the dangers posed by sharks and air travel, the risk of dying in an automobile accident is vastly greater. Yet I doubt you will lose any sleep over that possibility tonight.

We need to analyze and understand our fears. We need to put them into perspective and push aside the irrational fears. If we don't, we risk allowing them to keep us from our dreams.

Triathlete Evan Del Colle, whom I talked about earlier in this book, has a positive view on fear. According to Evan, "You have to realize that in the world there is a lot of fear of failure because people can't accept failure." Instead, Evan says, "I embrace failure, because when I fail, I know it's not going to happen again." Evan sees failure as his teacher, not as his enemy.

When it comes to the Iron-distance, I want you to respect it, but not to fear it. It is doable. Thousands have proven that already. Take all rational safety precautions, trust in your plan, and follow your plan one day at a time. Don't look too far down the road and don't allow irrational fears to curtail you.

Techniques for Controlling Your Thoughts

While I do not have a degree in psychology, the real-world experience I have gained out there in over thirty Iron-distance races is about as real as it gets. My opinions on the mental aspects of Iron-distance racing are based on my personal experience as an athlete and a coach.

Having said this, we need to make mental training part of our daily Iron-distance training—not something we revisit from time to time, but a key element we focus on every day. Following are two effective techniques for training yourself to control your thoughts. I have successfully employed these methods with dozens of athletes. I refer to them as "Get to That Point" and "You Believe What You Hear."

• "Get to That Point"

Create situations in your training where you "get to that point" at which you experience self-doubts and fear. Some of the best types of training sessions for this are the Long Runs and Long Rides, as well as the high-intensity runs and rides.

Perhaps you are 2 hours into a 3-hour ride and you find yourself doubting your ability to finish. Or suppose you are doing five 6-minute high-intensity runs, and after only the second one you start to doubt your ability to do three more.

In these moments of distress we experience mental challenges very similar to the ones we experience in an actual race. These moments provide us with two basic choices: We can give in to them, or we can challenge ourselves to mentally work through them. Obviously we want to do the latter and, further, we want to train ourselves over time to consistently do the latter. We want to build a mental pattern of not giving in.

How do we do this? First, when you "get to that point," try to relax. Mentally step away from your fears and self-doubts and look at them objectively. Remind yourself that these are normal feelings that virtually all endurance athletes experience, and also that they are temporary. Finally, realize that you have a unique opportunity to become mentally stronger. Consciously decide to hold on to it and take full advantage of it.

Play mental games to get through the discomfort. When I have self-doubts and am considering quitting, I count. That's right: I count. I promise myself that I will continue for a count of 100. I count right along with my breathing pattern. Each breath is one. When I get to 100, I make the exact same challenge to myself again. I agree to go on for 100 more breaths.

My commitment goes no further than the next 100 breaths, and I don't think beyond that point. But I find that each time I count to 100, I am able to agree to 100 more.

I utilized this technique when I ran the double marathon (52.4 miles) third day stage of the 2002 Ultraman World Championships. This stage takes place after 6.2 miles of ocean swimming and over 262 miles of cycling. At 36 miles into the double marathon, I began to doubt I could make it. I started to promise myself that I would run for only 100 breaths more, and then I would reconsider quitting. I kept running for 100 breaths. I kept making a new promise to myself.

Estimating that I take about 100 breaths every quarter mile, I figure I made over six thousand small promises to myself in those last 16 miles. Thanks to my mental training, all those little promises added up to an unforgettable personal victory.

- **"You Believe What You Hear"**

Most of us are raised to be modest. When someone pays us a compliment, we often feel uncomfortable. Instead of thanking the person for the compliment, many of us are conditioned to dismiss it. From childhood to adulthood, decade after decade, we condition ourselves to dismiss such compliments. "Oh, I'm not so fast . . . ," "My competitors must have been having a bad day . . . ," "I was just lucky . . . ," and so on.

The problem with all this politeness is that after hearing yourself say it for 30 years, you tend to believe it. You have talked yourself into it. You condition yourself to believe that you are not capable of achieving great things.

Learn to control your thoughts by learning to say "Thank you." It's as simple as that. By graciously accepting a compliment, we train ourselves to expect good things and a generally positive outcome. We want to train ourselves to believe that, sure, occasionally things don't work out, but most of the time we are successful—most of the time great things happen.

I am often reminded of a statement Lance Armstrong made after his recovery from cancer. "I now have two kinds of days," Lance said. "Good days and great days." This is the attitude we want to develop. Sure, everything doesn't always go your way, but something great lies just around the next corner. Train yourself every day to have this attitude.

In this next exercise, I challenge you to put the "You Believe What You Hear" concept into action for yourself. My challenge is in the form of a game. Try it out with the assistance of your spouse or a friend.

TAKE ACTION CHALLENGE:
THE POSITIVE AFFIRMATION GAME

The Positive Affirmation Game works particularly well when you make it an ongoing challenge between you and your spouse or a friend you spend a great deal of time with. Whenever you catch the other person in the game saying something negative about himself, the "punishment" is that he has to say something positive about himself aloud five times. He can say whatever he wants, but it must be true and he must say it like he means it. The game helps you discover how you talk negatively about yourself and how to overcome that tendency in your thinking.

Family Support

While you are the one making the choice to take on the Iron-distance challenge, those around you—your spouse, children, other family members, close friends—will also bear part of the burden, whether or not they are even asked. No matter how efficient you become with your training and time management, there will be some impact on your family as you train. As your training load increases, some family members may even resent what you have taken on. Remember, it may be your dream, but it is probably not theirs. Still, you need their support.

I encourage all athletes to conduct a "Family Meeting" when they decide to take on the Iron-distance. The Family Meeting can be an important part of the mental preparation needed both by the athlete and by his or her loved ones. This technique is highly recommended for all those training for an Iron-distance triathlon, especially those with important family and career responsibilities. You need to put your life in order to train for and successfully complete an Iron-distance triathlon.

What do I mean by a Family Meeting? Plan a time to discuss your Iron-distance plan with your spouse, children, and any other family members you regularly depend on. Be as honest as you can. Tell them about your dream. Let them know how important this goal is to you and why. Most importantly, ask them for their support. Ask them to be part of your team to achieve this goal.

This is so important. As you spend growing hours training and less time with them, you want them to feel that it is their goal too, and only with their support will you be able to achieve it.

Otherwise, they may begin to resent your time away from them and be less than fully supportive. They are too important to let this happen. You need their support and you need to share your dream with them.

As we saw earlier, Kathleen Hughes, a world-class Masters triathlete and mother of two preteen girls, says spousal support is one of the greatest factors in her success. When her husband, Jim, a busy attorney, first learned of her Iron-distance dream, he was very supportive. As with many who learn that a loved one has committed to take on the Iron-distance challenge, Jim felt that it was probably a onetime thing. She would take on this great challenge, but after she accomplished it she would return to normal life.

However, the Iron-distance experience changed Kathleen, just as it has changed virtually all who have accomplished it. Kathleen decided that Iron-distance racing would become a part of her life going forward. Jim embraced this, and became not only a great supporter of Kathleen's goal, but also a fan of her sport. Kathleen, who is now considered one of the best in the world in her age group, credits Jim for much of her success.

One of the good things about Iron-distance training is that it is fairly predictable. You will probably enter your race as much as a year in advance of the actual race date. You will know very early which weekends you need to keep free for training, and you can plan accordingly way in advance. If you follow one of the 30-week programs I present in this book, you will know your exact training time requirements for every day over the next seven months.

By having your Family Meeting early, you can get everybody involved and give them a good understanding of the training schedule. My experience has been that if you have this family meeting early and make your family understand how important this goal is to you, it is virtually always successful. The family pulls together for your goal. In many cases, the Ironman race and the training that preceded it become a great piece of family history and a fond memory.

I recommend a similar approach at work. Have a sit-down with your boss and possibly a separate meeting with some of your key coworkers who rely on you. Let them know you don't expect it to have any impact on your work, and you will of course use vacation time when you travel for the race itself, but also let them know how important this is to you, and ask for their patience and support, just in case you might be a little late for work someday, or a little grumpy one Monday morning following a long training weekend.

In my experience in the business world, this approach works great. Some bosses have become so inspired and impressed with you for taking on such a challenge that they almost insist you take some extra hours here and there when you need them.

My personal experience with Citigroup was extremely positive. They were always behind me and if I had to leave a little early or something one day, they were encouraging. It was a smart move too, because when I came back to the office after big races, I used to work extra long hours out of gratitude for their wonderful handling of the situation. To this day, I feel extreme loyalty to Citigroup for joining my team, just as I had joined their team.

Tip: *Encourage your family members to be a volunteer on race day. It's amazing how volunteering makes you feel a part of the race. Many volunteers are so moved by the experience, that they come back every year to do it again, and some even go on to become Ironmen themselves.*

The Importance of Mentors

Finding mentors is one of the most important steps to success. At the least, an effective mentor can eliminate years of trial and error and greatly accelerate your learning curve. At best, a mentor can change your life. Without a doubt, one good mentor can be all the difference between an average life and a truly extraordinary life.

While one good mentor is good, we can all benefit from many mentors, in many different parts of our lives—in athletics, career, marriage, parenting, and spirituality. We need to reach out to mentors continually and keep adding them to our team throughout our lives. I call this ongoing process "mentor gathering." It has been a core success technique for me. If you are pursuing a goal, I strongly encourage you to seek mentors.

Mentors can take many forms. They may range from a close personal coach (which I highly recommend, if you can afford this luxury), to an inspirational figure you never even meet. The key is that mentors help us move more quickly up the learning curve, avoid mistakes and setbacks, and eliminate the time-consuming process of trial and error.

By reading this book, you may consider me to be one of your mentors. If so, I am honored. It is one of the reasons I wrote this book. So many great people have helped me to succeed. In part I will repay my debt to them by writing this book. Someday, when you reach your Iron-distance goal, you will undoubtedly turn to others to help them achieve their dreams. After you achieve your dreams you will find, as I have, that true success comes when you help others to be successful. This is what mentoring is all about.

Why doesn't everyone seek out mentors? There are many reasons. For one, many people don't like to ask for directions. They like to "go it alone."

If you are like this, I encourage you to move beyond this self-imposed constraint. Mentoring is just too important to allow your ego to prevent you from experiencing it.

Some people do not seek mentors out of a fear of embarrassment. They fear rejection and shy away from even contacting potential mentors. Please work to get beyond this. Mentoring is key to achieving your dream.

Here are a few tips to help you find mentors:

- Mentors rarely find you. You need to be proactive to find them. Take action!

- One mentor is not enough. Build a team of several mentors for each area in which you want to improve (e.g., athletics, family, or career). Make "mentor gathering" an ongoing pursuit.

- A face-to-face relationship is preferred, but it is not always possible or necessary. You can have a long-distance mentor and stay in touch via telephone, email, or fax. Two of my best mentors over the years were Troy Jacobson and Karen Smyers. Both live a couple of states away, but while each was coaching me, we stayed in close weekly contact.

- Speaking of coaches, don't forget "mentors for hire." In many sports and other areas of interest, you can hire coaches and teachers with great experience and the ability to communicate their experience to you. While a full-time coach is expensive, online coaching can be very affordable.

- If a paid coach is still too expensive, consider clinics, camps, and workshops. In addition to having some intensive learning and training in your area of interest, you may very well identify potential mentors at these sessions. Have some fun too! Combine a clinic with a vacation. Go with a friend or make new ones.

- If a potential mentor ever does reject you, don't let it discourage you. Use it to fuel your competitive fires and to become even more determined to accomplish your goals. Just move on and find another mentor.

One final thought on mentors: Mentors do more than teach us skills, they motivate us by helping us believe in our ability to grow and improve. Become a mentor to someone else. True success comes when we give back to others and help them to achieve their goals.

TAKE ACTION CHALLENGE: MENTOR GATHERING

List the names of three mentors you currently have in each of the following three areas: athletics, family, and career.

Now go back and after each name write the approximate last date of contact with them. Now ask yourself the following questions:

How easy was it to come up with three names for each?

Has my contact with all of them been frequent and current?

Do their areas of expertise fully cover all of my desired areas of self-improvement?

The results of this exercise will help make it clear to you whether or not you are using your mentors effectively to achieve your goals. If you are less than fully satisfied with your result, use the mentor-gathering tips above to build up your personal team of mentors.

Overcoming Setbacks

Usually we first become aware of successful athletes after they have reached the peak of their game—the Olympics, the Tour de France, or some other world-class showcase event. We may be somewhat familiar with a couple of these athletes as they move up through the ranks in their sport, but for the most part we don't hear about them until they reach the top. Our first impression of them is therefore formed at a point in their careers when they are at their very best.

When we see these athletes for the first time performing at near-perfect levels, it may occur to us how "gifted" they are, that they are so lucky to be born with this natural ability. After all, they make it look so easy. The reality, however, is quite different from what it first appears to be. Reaching this point was far more difficult for them than we can see.

Was this athlete just born with such great talent that he/she was able to float through the first twenty-one years of her life and on to her destiny at the Olympics? In virtually all cases, the answer is no. More than likely, there were years of training, sacrifice, trial and error, and less than fully supportive people to deal with on their journeys. There were probably injuries and illnesses as well. These athletes encountered setbacks and obstacles along the way that at times severely threatened their chances of even continuing in their sport, let alone making it to the top.

Successful people in athletics, and life in general, are not those who have been so lucky as to never encounter a setback. They are people who, through whatever means—persistence, desire, strength of will—have overcome each setback along the way. Our success in athletics (or anything else) has less to do with whether or not we face setbacks than it does with how we deal with setbacks once we encounter them—and we will encounter them.

Triathlete Kathleen Hughes is an example of a top athlete who has developed techniques for successfully dealing with setbacks. When faced with an injury or a setback, Kathleen takes the attitude that, "I need to be bigger than the problem." Instead of denying or avoiding the issue, or wishing the situation were different than it is, she takes it head-on. Kathleen believes that the best course of action is to quickly accept the reality of the situation. Don't focus on where you wanted to be. Focus on where you are. As Kathleen puts it, "Live in the present and the future. Explore your options to maximize your comeback."

A couple years back, Kathleen had a plantar fasciitis flare-up that threatened her season. A doctor advised her that this type of foot injury requires complete rest from athletics. Kathleen considered this option, but she also considered pool running, some new stretching exercises, and some modifications to her training program, which emphasized more swimming and cycling. As it turned out, Kathleen's creativeness, positive attitude, and tenacity paid off. She went on to win several age-group victories in major races that year, as well as All American honors.

Psychologist and triathlete Pete Dominick stresses the importance of approaching setbacks with the right attitude. "Focus on how you can turn your setback into an opportunity. If you have an injury that prevents you from running, you may be able to use the time to improve your swim. If you can accomplish this, your performance may actually improve in the long run as a result of a setback." Pete also adds, "While we usually focus on preparing for our next big event, in times of setback it can be helpful to put our short-term goals into perspective, and focus on the journey and our overall lifelong goals."

There is no more amazing example of what an athlete's tenacity and determination can overcome than what Lance Armstrong has accomplished over the past several years. No matter what we face in the future, Lance has helped us all put setbacks into perspective. Surely the thought of quitting had to have entered Lance's mind at some point as he battled his illness, just as it does for most people when the situation looks bleak. However, Lance Armstrong not only beat incredible odds just to be able to race again, he took his performance to a new level.

We all have goals for athletics and life. On the way to those goals there will always be setbacks and obstacles that will challenge our resolve. Hang in there when times are tough. Remember what we have learned from the great ones: It truly is not what life does to us that will ultimately determine our success and happiness; it is how we handle what life does to us. Keep this in mind as you take your journey. I wish you the best in realizing your goals and dreams.

AN *IRONFIT* MOMENT

From out of the Darkness (written in 2002)
The following "IronFit Moment" is about an athlete I coached who taught me and many others about what it means to deal with setbacks and perseverance.

"She's out of the water!" I called to my wife. "Sarah is out of the water and she's going to make it!" My wife rushed into my office to find me following Ironman Florida in progress on the Internet.

She knew immediately what I was talking about: Triathlete Sarah Crewe was on her way to accomplishing something great—something that seemed impossible only a couple of months ago.

For someone like Sarah Crewe, completing the swim in an Ironman race may not seem like such a big deal. After all, both Sarah and her husband Patrick are veteran triathletes. In prior years, Sarah had conquered the Hawaii Ironman, Ironman Europe, Ironman Lanzarote, and many more of the sport's toughest tests. In the year 2000, however, things were very different.

It all started in January during a vacation in Hawaii. A devastating bike crash left Sarah with a shattered clavicle and scapula, along with several other related injuries. During emergency surgery, a titanium plate and eight screws were inserted in Sarah's shoulder. Her arm and shoulder were immobilized for over 8 weeks.

When Sarah's arm was finally "free to move," there wasn't much in the way of movement. She could lift her hand no more than an inch away from her thigh. Her shoulder was officially "frozen." As her training log would indicate one month later, Sarah went through a very tough time, both mentally and physically.

Sarah's training log entry on April 2, 2000: "After a month of rehab, I still cannot move my arm above my shoulder . . . yet. I go to physical therapy every other day, where the therapist 'tortures' me until I cry. My doctor says that it will be the better part of a year before I am back. I went through a tough mental spot a few weeks ago, and to cheer myself up I registered for Ironman Florida."

Despite the bleak outlook, Sarah kept battling to come back. In addition to the initial injuries, muscle imbalances developed, further complicating her recovery. There were many days when she feared she would never race again, and even if she did, it would only be as a shadow of her former self. Sarah kept pushing these thoughts aside, as she clung to the slim hope of returning to race Ironman Florida at the end of the year.

Sarah's training log entry on May 23, 2000: "I have a long way to go. Doc says a year. Therapy three times per week. Still I cannot swim, and my periformus is painful. I'm doing strength work to build up my atrophied muscles. As my physical therapist says, I'm a mess. This is definitely my off year, although I did sign up for Ironman Florida . . . we'll see."

As the weeks went by, Sarah made only small, incremental improvements. And even then there were continual setbacks. Often the thrill of a good day was followed by the letdown of a couple of bad days. Sarah gave herself mental pep talks several times each day, fighting to make it through the dark moments.

Finally a fork in the road approached—possibly a moment of truth. It was late August, a week before the withdrawal deadline for Ironman Florida. Sarah considered her options. There was a chance she could make it to the race. But in what kind of condition? Was it worth it to go through this pain any longer? Maybe she should drop out now and just write off the year 2000 and just try to forget it.

After a great deal of contemplation, the answer became clear. Sarah could still make it a year of great accomplishment . . . a year of personal victory. Sarah decided that she must define her own goal. Her goal would be to finish Ironman Florida in good health. Not to win her age group, not to set a personal best time at the Iron-distance. Only to finish in good health.

This was difficult for an Iron-distance veteran, but Sarah chose to define her own success. She wasn't going to focus on her past performances or how well she might have done without this setback. Accomplishing this goal would end the year on a high note. It would draw the line clearly between the injury of the past and the personal victories of the future.

The months of September and October were not easygoing. There was gradual progress, but also many more tough days. There were more setbacks, more self-doubt, more tears. But somehow Sarah kept moving forward, focused on her goal.

Well, Sarah did make it back to the Panama City beach on that November morning after her 2.4-mile swim. She then battled her way through 112 miles in the Florida heat and wind to a surprisingly fast bike split. And later that day, Sarah ran across the finish line after her marathon in good health, good spirits, and, yes, with her fastest Ironman time ever.

Sarah will remember this year—a year that might have been one of her darkest—as one of her greatest years, a year of overcoming seemingly unbeatable obstacles and, through her determination, achieving a great personal victory. When times seem to be at their darkest, remember Sarah Crewe's example. Reevaluate your goals and keep moving forward. No matter how small your progress may seem at times, the light ahead will be much closer than you think.

CHAPTER 16

Effective Goal Setting and Race Selection

"If you fail to plan, you plan to fail."

—Anonymous

Effective Goal Setting

Effective goal setting is a powerful tool in the pursuit of the Iron Dream. For the ultimate race, as well as for all of the training and preparation stages leading up to it, effective goal setting can provide both motivation and focus.

When athletes request my advice on how to improve their athletic performance, I often start by asking them the following two questions:

- Do you think that you are more likely to achieve your goals if you put them in writing? Most athletes answer "Yes."

- Do you have clearly defined goals and do you consistently record them in writing? Almost all athletes answer "No."

We all seem to believe that we can improve our athletic performance by establishing goals and writing them down. The question is why don't we?

To paraphrase Yogi Berra, "90% of success is half mental." While his remark was humorous, there is a point in it that applies to athletic competition. As important as physical skills are, it takes well-honed mental skills to achieve our fullest potential. Proper goal setting is one of the first steps to building a positive mental focus.

Why Goal Setting Is So Difficult

Let's get right to the heart of the issue. Setting goals is, at best, uncomfortable. By setting a goal, we establish a commitment. By establishing a commitment, we risk failure. Commitment. Failure. These are powerful words.

Why not keep our goals a little fuzzy? Isn't it safer just to say, "I will try to do my best"? Well sure, that approach is fine. After all, athletics are fun and we all enjoy them in different ways. Those who find the greatest fulfillment in improving their personal performances, however, must be prepared to leave their comfort zone. Instead of avoiding the fear of commitment and failure, try using it to your advantage. If you confront your fears and examine them, I think you will agree that the upside far outweighs the downside.

The following two points are "truths" for me and maybe you will find that they are "truths" for you as well:

- Fear of failure is a powerful motivator. It is up to you to decide if it is going to be a positive motivator or a negative one. You can choose to avoid fear or you can choose to channel it in a positive way.

- Fear of failure is taken too seriously. The reality is that nobody really cares about the finer points of your performance anyway. Your true friends and family want you to enjoy what you are doing. They respect you for your commitment and for the fact that you show up on race day and give it your best. Whether you are first across the finish line or 999th doesn't matter to them. The only one it really matters to is you.

I find that by reminding myself of these "truths" from time to time, I can keep the fear of failure in perspective.

I once tried to avoid the fear of failure by keeping my ever-changing goals to myself and rarely declaring them in writing. I came to realize this was not effective goal setting. After years of slow progress, I started experimenting with writing goals in my training log. At first these were fuzzy goals like, "improve on my best performances from last year." Over time, however, I started to commit to more specific goals. Not only did I start to see better results, I began to enjoy my sport more and more. The further I took goal setting, the more I enjoyed it and the better my performances became.

Setting and Committing to Your Goals

At the beginning of the season, establish specific goals for your races and write them down. Most training logs have calendars and note pages in the back where you can do this. Be specific. For each of your races, record an overall time goal, e.g., complete Ironman Lake Placid in under 11 hours. Then record all three targeted splits, e.g., swim 1:05, bike 5:45, run 4:09. Also record your place goal, e.g., top ten in my age group. Being this specific will help you to focus. Finally, your goals should be "stretch goals." They should be challenging but not impossible to achieve.

Once I was convinced that by committing myself to my goals I was more likely to achieve them, I began experimenting with ways of taking my commitment to a higher level. My most successful method to date is what I call "posting goals." I actually create a sign with the name of my next race at the top, my splits and my overall time in the middle, and my desired placing at the bottom. I then post one copy of the sign on the mirror of my bathroom (it's the first thing I see every morning when I turn on the light), one copy

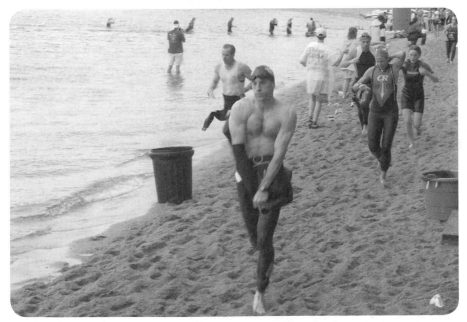

Peter Hyland, married, father, chemist . . . Iron-distance triathlete.
Photo Credit: Allison Hyland.

on the wall in front of my cycling trainer, and one copy in my office. This may sound like overkill, but try it. It really works.

LAKE PLACID IRONMAN
SUB 11:00 HRS

SWIM	BIKE	RUN
1:05	5:45	4:09

TOP TEN AGE GROUP

I find that two interesting things happen when you post your goals. First, it's a commitment. Your goals are not hidden away in the back of your training log. They are out in the open in black and white. Anyone who visits your home or office is likely to ask you to explain your poster. Every time you explain what it is, you restate your commitment—"Oh that? That's my goal for my next race." The more people you tell your goal to, the more committed to it you become.

Another interesting result I have noticed is that over the several weeks that my sign is posted, I gradually feel that my goals are more and more achievable. There have been times when I felt a little embarrassed at first because the goal seemed to be too unbelievable. By the time of the actual race, however, I felt the goal was too easy. By looking at my goal every day, by thinking about it again and again, by visualizing myself achieving it, I eventually accepted it to the point where I would show up on race day fully convinced that I would achieve that performance.

I have since experimented with posting more ambitious goals and have had corresponding success. I used to "low ball" my goals to my family and friends, trying to avoid the added pressure of their expectations. I would say things like, "Oh, I'll be happy with a place in the top ten." The truth was I wanted to win and I honestly believed I had a shot at it.

Well, no more low balling. I tell anyone who asks specifically what my goal is and sometimes I even let him know that I would appreciate his or her help in achieving it. In a sense, I make my goal, their goal.

The following is a summary of the key steps in maximizing the power of effective goal setting:

- Establish specific goals for your overall racing season and for each individual race.

- Make your goals as quantifiable as possible (e.g., times, places, splits, etc.).

- Record your goals in writing and review them frequently.

- Post your goals for your next race in places where you (and others) will see them frequently. Think about them every day and visualize yourself achieving them.

- Express your goals honestly to your coach, friends, and family.

The mental aspect in sports is crucial. Training your mind is as important as training your body. Effective goal setting is a key ingredient to healthy motivation and successful racing. I hope the above ideas will contribute to your success and enjoyment of the sport.

In this next exercise I challenge you to establish effective goals and then use the "Post Your Goals" technique to commit to and believe in these goals.

TAKE ACTION CHALLENGE: POSTING YOUR GOALS

Post your goals! Right now, write down on a piece of paper your specific goals for the Iron-distance, following the guidelines above. Post at least one copy in a place where you will see it at least every morning. When you see your posted goals for the first time each morning, reaffirm your commitment to yourself by reading them aloud.

Race Selection

All Iron-distance races are not the same. They may all be the same distance, but topography, climate, altitude, and atmosphere differ from race to race. Some race directors go out of their way to be open and supportive for first timers; other races have a highly competitive atmosphere and focus more on the professionals and elite age groupers. Some races have fewer than 100 competitors, some have over 2,000. Some favor swimmers, some cyclists, and some runners.

An important consideration in your first Iron-distance triathlon is race selection. Choosing the right race can have a big effect on how successful you are in achieving your goals.

Many of us first learned about Iron-distance racing by seeing the Hawaii Ironman on television. It strikes a chord with so many people. For many, it's the most amazing accomplishment they can imagine. For this reason, it is no wonder that many want their first Iron-distance—sometimes even their first triathlon!—to be the Hawaii Ironman. This is possible (see below) but unlikely. My advice is to make the Hawaii Ironman a long-term goal. Don't hold off racing your first Iron-distance triathlon for several years waiting for the opportunity.

Here's the good news: Most of the Ironman-distance races out there are great. The Iron-distance experience is now offered in many different forms and in many different places. I have raced all around the world, in the biggest and the smallest races, and virtually every one of them was magnificent. My experiences from all of them were so memorable.

In fact, my wife often jokes with me that I fall in love with every Iron-distance location I visit. I guess it's such a wonderful and emotional experience, and the people are always so warm and supportive, that I form a deep attachment to the race, the people, and the state or country where it takes place.

So go ahead, set your long-term sights on Hawaii. I would love every triathlete to have the experience of racing in Hawaii someday. But don't let that hold up your first Iron-distance triathlon. Find a race that's right for you, do the right preparation, and go have the magnificent Iron-distance experience.

Finding the Best Race for You

When selecting your first race, think about what type of environment will be most conducive to you accomplishing your goal.

Consider the atmosphere of the race. What will motivate you the most? Will you be motivated by racing with some of the stars of the sport, or might you find this a little intimidating for your first race? Perhaps a race with many first-time Ironmen like you might feel more supportive.

Consider the date of the race and how that fits into your career and family life schedule. Based on the training schedules presented in Chapter 7, you can easily determine when the peak training periods are least likely to interfere with other responsibilities.

Consider the size of the race. In a big race, with 2,000 competitors, you are likely to find other athletes to run with and motivate you through those last tough miles. On the other hand, you may find solitude in a less crowded race of only a few hundred.

Other considerations may include matching your personal strengths and weaknesses to the course itself. For example, Ironman Florida has a pancake-flat bike and run course, but has a sometimes challenging ocean swim, depending on conditions. If your strength is the swim and you're weaker in either the bike or the run, this may be the perfect course for you. If it's the other way around (i.e., you are a weak swimmer and a strong cyclist or runner), this course may not be best suited for you.

Consider the climate. Do you prefer competing where it's cool or where it's hot? Check the race's Web site to see what the expected weather will be like on race day. Also consider altitude. If you live and train at sea level, you are likely to race best at a sea-level competition.

Virtually all Iron-distance triathlons, with the exception of Hawaii itself, allow wetsuits, which is a big asset for weaker swimmers.

Don't forget to plan early. Many of the major Iron-distance races, including most of the World Triathlon Corporation–affiliated races in North America, fill up very quickly, even though they all have field limits of around 2,500 athletes. You may have to be willing to commit to these races up to a year in advance.

It should be noted, however, that all have a withdrawal deadline, which allows you to get a portion of your entry fee back if you have a change in plans and need to withdraw.

In addition to the Hawaii Ironman World Championships, there are over twenty Iron-distance races to choose from affiliated with the World Triathlon Corporation and dozens and dozens of independent races around the world, which are all at the same Iron-distance, though not connected with the World Triathlon Corporation.

Hawaii Ironman World Championships

First, let's start with a look at the "Big Kahuna." The Hawaii Ironman celebrated its thirtieth anniversary in 2008. What can I say about this race? For triathletes, the Kona course is sacred ground. This is the heart and soul of our sport and virtually every multisport athlete wants to do this race, at least at some point.

Needless to say, this is one tough race to win entry to. That's right . . . win. There are over 1,800 entry slots available to be won at one of the many World Triathlon Corporation races held around the world. Usually you need to finish at or very near the top of your age group in one of these races to secure one of the coveted slots. There are also a small number of lottery slots offered each year. The Ironman lottery is held early in the year and thousands participate.

The Hawaii course is one of the most challenging of all of the Ironmans. The severe heat, high winds, non-wetsuit ocean swim, deceptive elevations, and fierce competition combine to earn this race's reputation as the toughest one-day endurance challenge in the world. There are pretty much only tough days and tougher days in this race.

Many joke that they worked so hard and so long to get to Hawaii, and then two hours into the race they started to wonder why. But that's what makes it so great. It's the challenge it offers and its unpredictability that makes it the race we all want to do.

Should this be your first Iron-distance race? As I mentioned above, probably not. Of course, if you win a lottery slot on your first try, you may not be able to refuse the opportunity. But in general, I would pick one of the other great races for your first Iron-distance experience.

World Triathlon Corporation (WTC)–Affiliated Races

The first place to look for a great Ironman race in the United States and Canada is among the WTC-affiliated races.

Without exaggeration, all of these races are excellent and set the standard for presenting top quality events.

In fact, if you want to do one of these races, you better make your plans early. In most cases entry slots are offered one year in advance, and most of these races sell out in a matter of hours.

Below are brief reviews of some of the WTC-affiliated races I am particularly fond of. I am going to dispense with telling you which ones are great, because they are all great!

• Ironman USA Lake Placid

This extremely popular Northeastern race started in 1999. Lake Placid is the perfect host. It is breathtakingly beautiful and, having hosted both the 1932 and 1980 Olympics, it has a rich athletic history.

The wetsuit swim includes two laps of the calm and pristine Mirror Lake. The super-challenging hills and descents of the two-lap bike course make this a "cyclist's Ironman." The challenge of the bike course makes the moderate hills of the two-lap run course feel much bigger than they really are.

Another factor to consider is competitiveness. This varies from age group to age group, but in general I would rank Lake Placid as one of the most competitive of the WTC-affiliated races. If you are shooting to win one of the coveted Hawaii Ironman entry slots, this is a factor you may want to consider.

• Ironman Canada

When I think of Ironman Canada, I immediately think of the warmth and commitment of the Penticton community. This beautiful town embraces the Ironman race like no other.

The swim, for which wetsuits are allowed, is in a cool glacier lake. Like the Lake Placid race, I would rate this as more of a "cyclist's race." One climb is about 7 miles in length. The challenging climbs of the bike course will make the "rollers" on the run course seem like serious hills.

Canada is one of the great triathlon countries so, as mentioned above, you can count on a competitive race. There will be plenty of talent in every age group.

Another factor to consider is this race's close proximity to the date of the Hawaii Ironman. It is likely to fall only about 6 or 7 weeks before Hawaii. If you are looking for a Hawaii qualifying opportunity, that is something to consider.

- **Ironman Wisconsin**

This Midwest addition was added in 2002 and sold out in its very first year. Madison is another great location. The WTC knows how to pick just the right kind of community to put on a world-class event.

Ironman qualifying slots won in this September race are for the Hawaii Ironman in the following October, 13 months away. Since it's only 1 month before Hawaii, however, those already racing Hawaii are likely to skip this race. This may afford an excellent opportunity to win a qualifying slot for the following year.

- **Ironman Florida**

Fast! That's what I think of when I think of the Southern edition, which began in 1999. While the seas in the Gulf can vary from calm to challenging, once you are out of the water, everything is flat and super-fast. This is a personal record course all the way. This is also an excellent race for a first timer.

Some feel that this is a particularly good opportunity to qualify for Hawaii, because it usually falls shortly after Hawaii. The theory goes that most of the top people will race in Hawaii and will not be racing again so soon, and if they do they won't be on their game. While this is true—few athletes do both races in a given year—this race always seems to be very competitive, with plenty of outstanding performances.

Independent Races

You may want to consider one of the independent races for your first Iron-distance triathlon. That's what I did, and it worked out well for me. There are no Hawaii Ironman qualifying slots to win, but these races are usually much less expensive and easier to enter.

Following is a list of six of the independent triathlons raced at the Iron-distance, and my thoughts on some of the ones I am most familiar with.

- Vineman Triathlon—Santa Rosa, CA

- Esprit Triathlon—Montreal, Canada

- Challenge Roth—Roth, Germany

- Duke Blue Devil Triathlon—Durham, NC

- Great Floridian Triathlon—Clermont, FL

- Chesapeake Man Ultra Distance Triathlon—Cambridge, MD

Vineman Triathlon

The Vineman Triathlon is based in Santa Rosa, California and is usually scheduled for August. It has some wonderful aspects, including a beautiful course winding through the wine country of Northern California.

The race usually has only about 300 to 500 competitors, so you don't have the crowded swim start that you find at most races. What's more, the race management prides themselves on the family atmosphere of the race and they deliver. It is a very supportive and nonthreatening environment, which can be just the right thing for many first-time Iron-distance competitors.

Here's a tip: Go for a little wine tasting the day after the race. It does wonders for those sore muscles!

Great Floridian Triathlon

Another great race for a first-time Iron-distance is the Great Floridian Triathlon in Clermont, Florida (near Orlando). Because it is held every year around the same time as Hawaii, this race is free from most of the hard-core Iron-distance competitors.

The event has great organization, friendly management, and supportive volunteers. Though it has a fairly big field, usually around 1,000, it maintains the feel of smaller races like Vineman and Esprit.

Swim times tend to be very fast on this course, while the hot rolling bike course tends to be slow.

It's also a great family race. After your kids watch you achieve your Iron-dream, you can thank them for their support with a trip to nearby Disney

World. This can be a great way to sell the whole Iron-distance concept to your loved ones in your Family Meeting.

- **Esprit Triathlon**

Another good low-key race is the Esprit Triathlon, which takes place in September at the site of the 1976 Olympics in Montreal. It too has a supportive and nonthreatening feel.

The wetsuit swim is in the Olympic rowing basin, which allows plenty of room to spread out. One of the really interesting features of this race is a criterion-style bike course; in other words, it's a "lap course." The bike segment calls for about forty-two laps of a Formula One race car circuit. Then the run is about nine laps around the Olympic rowing basin. The entire course is flat and doesn't favor any one sport over another.

Esprit holds a special place in my heart, because it was my first Iron-distance race. I enjoyed this race—in fact I have raced it three times—but it may not be for everyone. Some may find it monotonous. The upside for the first timer is that your friends and family can watch and cheer you on through the entire race. This kind of ongoing personal attention from loved ones can be a great confidence builder.

CHAPTER 17

Maintaining Good Health

"Give them great meals of beef and iron
and steel, they will eat like wolves and
fight like devils."

—William Shakespeare, King Henry V

Injuries are common in all athletics, and unfortunately triathlon is no exception. It can be so frustrating when injuries delay us from achieving our goals, especially when they are injuries that can be avoided.

I often see athletes making the mistake of not promptly addressing injuries in their early stages. They ignore them and hope the injuries will get better on their own. Sometimes this works (if you're lucky), but many injuries linger, grow worse, and then require long recuperation periods. I suggest that you err in the direction of caution and early treatment.

Injury Prevention and Care

First, anyone starting to train for an Iron-distance triathlon should have a complete physical with a qualified medical professional. You should advise your doctor of exactly what you plan to do and make sure that he or she confirms that it is safe for you to take on this physical challenge. Return for a complete physical every year, and always make sure your doctor knows exactly what type of training and racing you are involved in.

Second, you should be proactive about aches, pains, and other problems that may arise. Don't delay. Consult a doctor about any of these issues immediately and solicit good advice on how to deal with them.

Don't rely on the advice of a well-intentioned friend or training partner. It's not worth the risk. Always get the advice of a qualified professional. This

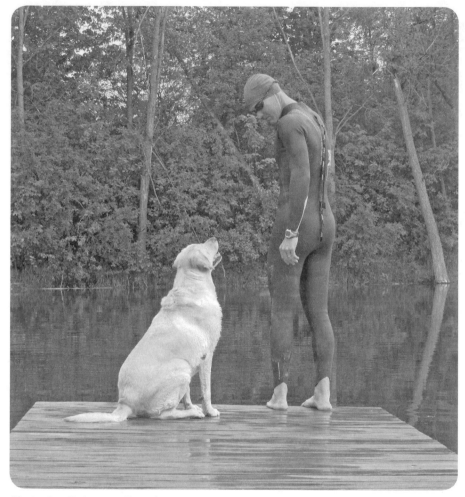

Photo Credit: Lynn Kellogg/www.trilifephotos.com.

may take a little time and cost a little money in the short run, but it will be well worth it in the long run.

In addition to the annual check-up with your primary physician, I also encourage you to put together a complete team of medical professionals with all of the specialties Iron-distance triathletes tend to require from time to time. It's best to have these individuals identified in advance, so you can act quickly when a need arises.

Your medical team may include your primary doctor, a sports podiatrist, an Active Release Therapy provider, an orthopedic surgeon, and a physical therapist. Your team might also include other health professionals for particular needs. For example, my team includes a dermatologist, as I have had occurrences of basal cell skin cancer in the past.

When I have a health issue of any type, I immediately go to the health care provider on my team who is best suited to deal with the problem. This way I am able to resolve small issues before they have a chance to become large issues, and thus maintain great consistency in training year after year.

How can you assemble a team of health care providers? Ask around for recommendations from people in the know. Triathlon clubs, multisport coaches, and other triathletes are usually the best sources.

You always want to identify health problems early and put in place the appropriate recovery plan as soon as possible. If this means missing a race in the short term, that's unfortunate, but in the long term there's always another race. After all, we want to be athletes for life.

In the following section, I will highlight Active Release Technique, which has recently grown to become one of the most helpful and popular means of health maintenance for triathletes.

Active Release Technique

Active Release Technique (ART) is a relatively new soft tissue approach for treating problems resulting from injury to over-used muscles. ART has been so helpful for triathletes; it's now common to see ART providers working with athletes at many Iron-distance events.

ART was developed by P. Michael Leahy, DC, CCSP, who noticed that his patients' symptoms seemed to be related to changes in their soft tissues that could be felt by hand. By observing how muscles, fascia, tendons, ligaments and nerves responded to different types of work, Dr. Leahy was able to consistently resolve many of his patients' problems.

Dr. John M. Schneider is a leading instructor for ART. He originally completed an internship with Dr. Leahy, and wrote "Active Release Techniques for the Cervical Spine in Conservative Management of Cervical Spine Syndromes," with Dr. Leahy. Dr. Schneider is currently a consultant for teams in the NFL, NHL, Major League Baseball and Major League Soccer.

He also treats a variety of athletes including elite triathletes, world-class sprinters, and professional wrestlers in the WWE.

In the following section, Dr. Schneider presents what he has found to be the most common triathlon-related injuries and how best to deal with them.

AN *IRONFIT* MOMENT

Dr. John Schneider on Active Release Technique (ART)

The world of triathlon is growing rapidly every year. With the increase in athletes, there is an increase in the number of injuries. Triathletes have many common injuries, and they can happen to everyone from the casual beginner to elite professionals. Many of these injuries are to the soft-tissue system—muscles, tendons, ligaments, fascia, and nerves. Many of these injuries are cumulative. That is not to say that traumatic injuries do not happen, but it is the overuse injuries that we are concerned with in this section.

If we are to understand these injuries, we must first understand how they happen. There are three types of soft-tissue injuries: acute, constant-pressure or tension injuries, and repetitive motion injuries. An acute injury is a result of direct trauma to the area, for example, a sprained ankle. A constant-pressure or tension injury is the result of sustained contraction or tension placed on an area. An example of this would be the tension placed upon the body from sitting with poor posture for extended periods of time. A repetitive-motion injury, which is the focus of this discussion, is a result of repeatedly doing a specific motion.

Repetitive-motion injuries are the most common injuries seen in the triathlon world. To understand these injuries we need a way to describe or quantify the amount of insult to the tissue. We use the Law of Repetitive Motion:

$$\text{INSULT to TISSUE} = \frac{\text{Number of Repetitions Performed} \times \text{Force of each Repetition}}{\text{Range of Motion of Repetition} \times \text{Relaxation} \times \text{Time of Repetition}}$$

For example, a marathon runner would take a large number of steps (Repetitions). He would use a moderate amount of force for each step, and the range of each step would be short. The relaxation between each step would be very short if the runner did not stop during the run. This would lead to a big insult to the soft tissue. Compare this to someone running a 100-meter sprint. The amount of steps the sprinter would take would be very small. The force of each repetition would be very large. The range of motion would be larger than that of the marathoner. The relaxation time would also be very small. This would lead to a much smaller insult to the tissue due to the significant difference in the amount of repetitions the marathon runner would take. The marathon runner would be more likely to get a repetitive motion injury; the sprinter would be more likely to get an acute injury. Now that we have an understanding that repetitive motion can be a large insult to tissue, let us see how this affects the triathlete.

Soft-tissue injury research in the last twenty years has changed the way we look at these injuries. The medical community believed soft-tissue injuries only happened in a traumatic situation such as a sprained ankle. The ankle injury would eventually heal, with scar tissue replacing the injured tissue. Research has shown that these repetitive-motion injuries can have the same effect on the soft tissue, with scar tissue accumulating within the tissue. This buildup of scar tissue diminishes the soft tissue's ability to do its job, whether that job is contraction of a muscle or a ligament providing stability. The cumulative-injury cycle demonstrates how the soft tissue responds to different stresses placed upon it. The cycle has three starting points depending on the injury. Each factor causes the next one in the cycle, which continually feeds the next part of the cycle.

For example, the repetitive-motion injury enters the cycle as weak and tense tissue. This leads to increased friction, pressure, and tension within the tissue. Next, the cycle enters either the inflammatory segment of the cycle, or if the injury is serious, the chronic segment. A newer injury leads to a tear or crush of the tissue. This leads to inflammation, and then adhesion and fibrosis takes place. Then the tissue gets weaker and the tension increases, which feeds into the friction, pressure, and tension part of the cycle—and the vicious cycle feeds itself until the cycle is broken. An acute injury enters the cycle in the tear or crush portion of the cycle. This leads to inflammation, adhesion and fibrosis, which weakens the tissue. If the injury heals properly, the cycle stops here, but if the injury does not recover properly then it continues down the chronic part of the cycle and along the same path of the repetitive-motion injury.

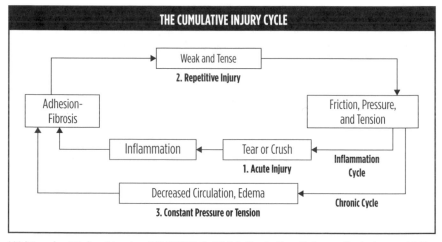

Written by Michael Leahy, DC CCSP. © 2000 By Active Release Techniques, LLC. All Rights Reserved.

Repetitive-motion injuries have specific areas that need to be addressed. The first is determining what tissue is injured. The next area is learning what caused the tissue to fail or get injured. The final step is determining what can be done to correct and prevent the injury recurring. We have already discussed the Law of Repetitive Motion and the Cumulative Injury Cycle. These two tools will help us identify the cause and response of the body. The correction of the problem can be a very simple answer, such as changing running shoes, changing training procedures, or correcting of the setup on your bike. For more complex problems where treatment is necessary Active Release Techniques is a popular choice for triathletes to fix their athletic injuries.

Active Release Techniques (ART) is a hands-on soft tissue management system that allows the practitioner to diagnose and treat soft tissue injuries. It is a process where all types of injuries can be treated—from the acute to the most chronic injuries. Soft tissue that has not properly healed or been treated will have changes that will affect the ability of the tissue to perform correctly, and will limit the athlete's ability to perform at his or her highest level. ART is used not only to treat soft-tissue injuries but to improve the performance of the athlete. By identifying specific biomechanical problems, a trained ART biomechanical practitioner can eliminate faults that can cause the athlete to waste energy and hinder ease of movement. Many times these biomechanical problems are the cause of repetitive-motion injuries. The body has to compensate around these problems and this causes tissue to be used in ways that it is not intended to be used. This leads to excessive stress or load placed upon this tissue and eventual failure of the tissue. This is where it enters the Cumulative Injury Cycle and the whole cascade of events occurs.

Triathletes have very specific injuries due to the nature of the sport, which all emphasize different parts of the body and therefore potentially lead to injury. Training for the swim portion places tremendous stress upon the shoulder. Training for the bike portion of the triathlon places a high demand of the hip and lower back. Training for the running portion of the race places a heavy burden on the athletes' knees. This discussion cannot go through every injury that a triathlete could encounter but we will go over three common injuries.

The swim portion of the triathlon places a high demand upon the shoulder. Swimmer's shoulder is a common term for shoulder impingement syndrome. This is where the rotator cuff of the shoulder is pinched and irritated when the athlete reaches over their head. If the injury is severe enough a tear of the rotator cuff is possible. Swimming for long periods of time can cause the soft tissue to fatigue and eventually fail. There can be many common causes

for this injury. Technique plays an important role in the development of repetitive motion injuries. Improper technique will cause
the athlete to recruit muscles incorrectly. This will stress these
muscles and muscular imbalances will occur. These muscle imbalances cause certain muscles to become very tight and other muscles to become inhibited from working properly. Common muscles
that become very tight are: the pectorals, the latissimus dorsi, the
upper trapezius, the levator scapulae, and the subscapularis. The
muscles that become inhibited are: the lower trapezius, the ser-
ratus anterior, the infraspinatus and the teres minor. Essentially the
prime movers of the shoulder in the swimming motion get over
developed and the stabilizing muscles of the shoulder blade get
inhibited. The end result of this imbalance is the supraspinatus
muscle of the rotator cuff gets pinched and inflamed. Swimming
technique is vital in placing the least amount of stress upon the
shoulder. Proper stretching and warming up of the prime movers
is important. Exercises directed towards strengthening the rotator
cuff and scapular stabilizers will help keep the balance between
prime mover and stabilizers. If the problem still exists, treatment of
these muscles with ART will improve the function and remove the
scar tissue that affects the muscles.

The bike portion of the triathlon places a high demand upon
both the hip and lower back. The hips and lower back regions
must work together as a unit for proper function to happen. Lower
back pain is very common for cyclists. Many times the setup of the
bike for a cyclist is the culprit. If the bike is not properly fitted for
the rider, biomechanical stress is placed on the rider for excessive
periods of time and many repetitions. This will lead to the soft tissue fatigue and failure. Common muscles that get tight are: the
psoas (or hip flexor), the adductors (or groin), the hamstrings,
and the quadriceps. Muscles of the lower back such as the erec-
tors and quadratus lumborum get compromised from the excessive time the cyclist stays in a bent over position. Low back pain
becomes evident in the transition from cycling to running. Cycling
places a high demand on the hip flexors. This causes them to get
excessively tight. When the triathlete begins to run he or she goes

from a forward flexed position (bent over) to an upright position of running. The hip flexors when tight will pull the lower back forward, creating a jamming of the joints of the lower back. It can be a few miles into the race before the hip flexors finally loosen up and allow the runner to move easier. Prevention of this problem begins with proper setup. Once that has been checked, stretching of the hip flexors, quadriceps, hamstrings, adductors, piriformis, and lower back will aid in eliminating the muscular imbalances.

The running portion of the race is very important. This is the most problematic of the three. Many injuries can happen to a runner. Since the run portion of the race is last, the athlete is the most fatigued and the risk of injury is the highest. Injuries from plantar fasciitis to hip injuries are all quite common. Illiotibial band syndrome (ITB syndrome) is one of the most common injuries for all runners. There are many things that can cause ITB syndrome. One of the most important areas to address is the hip. If the hip is not functioning correctly the runner's center of gravity will shift more to one side than the other. The side that is affected is usually on the side of hip dysfunction. Commonly tight muscles are: the tensor fascia lata (TFL), the piriformis, the gluteus medius, the adductors, the hamstrings, and the psoas or hip flexor. The balance between the gluteus medius and the adductors is what keeps the runner from falling over while standing on one leg. The function of the foot is very important with ITB syndrome. If someone is very flat footed, also known as pronation, the leg is placed in a position that is not biomechanically efficient and places a twisting force upon the ITB. If this stress is continued long enough, inflammation occurs and the cumulative-injury cycle takes over. Proper stretching of the psoas, piriformis, gluts, hamstring, and adductors are very important. Strengthening of the gluteus medius is also very important. Choice of shoes can play a role in what happens to the kinematics of the leg. If you are a pronator and use shoes that do not correct for this, the knee will be placed into internal rotation and the ITB will be stressed. Orthotics are inserts placed into your running shoes that help with stabilizing your feet. This helps with the chain reactions of muscular contractions that give the leg its stability. If these simple interventions do not correct the injury, treatment of the soft tissue and strengthening will be necessary.

Triathlons place a high demand on the athlete's body. Each triathlon leg has its own specific injuries, and a good understanding of the biomechanics of each sport is necessary in treating triathletes. The triathlon distance, whether it is a sprint triathlon or Iron-distance, can also determine the potential injuries. Sprint triathlons are more ballistic in movement compared with the endurance and survival of an Iron-distance race. Each athlete must be evaluated individually to determine the specifics of each condition. Many times it is the understanding of how the injury took place that will lead to the correction and resolution of the problem.

Sleep

As I have stressed throughout this book, effective time management is one of the pillars of Iron-distance success. When highly motivated people, often with families and careers, take on the Ironman challenge, they usually strive to eliminate unnecessary time-consuming activities from their schedules. Often sleep is included in this category. This is a mistake.

I urge you to get as much sleep as possible. Adequate sleep keeps you healthy and allows your body to absorb the benefits of training without becoming worn down. As I have said earlier, the way to build fitness efficiently is to combine just the right blend of athletic stress with rest.

How much sleep is needed? It really depends on the person. The gold standard is 8 hours, but very few busy athletes seem to get this much, especially during the week. Depending on the person, 7 hours may be a more realistic target to shoot for. Once the average slips below 6 hours, however, most athletes are slipping into the danger zone: They are not fully recovering from the stress of training and risking illness or injury as a result.

As seen in some of the profiles presented earlier, many athletes have tricks for increasing their amount of sleep time. Some athletes lay out their clothes and set up their equipment the night before early morning training sessions, and then go to bed as early as possible. Many athletes nap during the day. One of our profiled athletes naps on the train or bus during his commute to work. If you drive to work, perhaps you can find a public transportation alternative that will allow you to take advantage of this approach. Depending on your work situation, you might be able to take a short nap at lunch, or some other break during the day. It is well worth taking your sleep seriously and working to maximize this important element of training.

Finally, if you feel extremely tired and not up to training, this is the perfect time to take a rest. If you are run down you will derive little benefit from training and you risk illness or injury. Do the smart thing: Take a day off and get a solid 8 hours of sleep. It is probably what your body needs. Then come back refreshed and healthy and put in solid training sessions for the remainder of the week.

CHAPTER 18

Healthy Eating for Endurance Athletes

"To eat is a necessity, but to eat
intelligently is an art."

—François de La Rochefoucauld

Got Married . . . Lost Forty Pounds

When I married Melanie twenty years ago, I was a fairly athletic 6'1" and 200 pounds. The extent of my weekly fitness routine included strength training with free weights three times a week and singles tennis three to four times a week. I ate pretty much whatever I wanted, when I wanted, and while no one would have called me fat, I was definitely carrying around more bulk than was optimal.

Melanie quickly changed all that once we were married. First, she reconnected me with my love for endurance sports, and second, she changed the way I ate. Not only did this change my body, it changed my life.

My current weight is about 160 pounds, and it has been that for at least the past twelve years. In fact it's rarely been more than a few pounds above or below that number over that time period—maybe a few pounds less right before a major race and a few pounds more in the off-season around the holidays.

While I frequently like to joke that I am the only man in America that got married and lost over forty pounds, it sure didn't happen how many people would guess it happened. The first thing most people say is something like, "Wow, forty pounds, what diet did you use?" Well the truth is, I never used any diet. In fact I lost the weight so gradually over a seven-year period, I never even felt like I was losing weight. There was never a month where I dropped even two or three pounds. It was all much more subtle than that.

Mine was a lifestyle change through a reconnection with endurance sports and a more healthy view of food as fuel for my body.

Due to my new "way of eating" and endurance training, very gradually and naturally I lost forty pounds over seven years. And what's really amazing is that once I got down around 160, my body stopped losing weight and started maintaining it at that level without my making any changes at all. It's almost like this really cool balance was achieved. By eating healthfully and training properly, my body just naturally assumed its optimal weight over seven years.

Now there, my body merely continues to maintain the balance. Not only does it feel like the right weight for me, but I perform better athletically at this weight and my cholesterol, blood pressure, and other vital signs are all better than ever. Those added bonuses were never really the goal, but they are a welcome side effect.

Because of my personal experience with weight loss, and my belief in being healthy and achieving a natural balance in all areas of life, I am not a big fan of the various diets out there. They mostly seem to have a short-term focus, and at some point the dieter returns to his or her same old ways and same old weight—or even heavier. One possible exception may be the Weight Watchers program, because it teaches individuals to eat real food in proper portions and in real-life situations.

If you are committed to being healthy and fit for life, the optimal path is to find the proper balance of nutrition and training that will allow you to be the athlete and healthy person you were meant to be.

While we may not want to admit it, leaner is usually faster. It's a simple matter of power-to-weight. All else being equal, if we have less weight to carry, we can move more quickly at the same level of effort. Sure, an athlete could take this to an extreme and get so thin that he or she becomes unhealthy and weak by losing muscle mass. There will always be some people who, for whatever reason, take a good thing too far. But generally our lightest healthy weight is usually our fastest weight.

Before starting any diet or nutrition plan, I encourage you to seek the advice of a competent nutrition expert. Let me say right up front that I am not a nutrition expert and I have no certifications in this field. What I talk about in this chapter is based on my personal experience with my own training and nutrition and feedback I have received from the hundreds of athletes I have worked with over the past decades. So please consider what I have to say, but before starting your own plan, get guidance from a certified professional.

At the end of this chapter, I list several free Web sites that can be very helpful in planning the best nutritional approach for you.

Six Small Meals

You already know a great deal about how I train, but how did I change my eating habits, which led to my gradual weight loss? Here's the quick answer: I ate six small meals every day.

That's right. I got away from the usual and traditional three-square-meals-a-day approach and started eating more frequently. Instead of three big meals averaging over 1,000 calories each (plus additional snacking in between), I started consuming six smaller meals averaging more like 600 calories each.

I discovered the first of many positives to this approach: My energy level was better throughout the day than ever before. It felt like I was more gradually giving my body calories over a longer period of time, and as a result it felt like the energy was always present when I needed it. Instead of periods of high energy and low energy, my energy level felt more constant and consistent throughout the day. This approach felt natural to me as soon as I began it, and it continues to feel that way today. When I want to train . . . I feel better physical energy. When I want to work . . . I feel mental energy. When I want to take my dogs for a run through the woods I am good to go.

How do we arrange the six small meals? Let's look at them as three mini meals and three big snacks. Here's an example of how it might work:

5:00 a.m. Wake up; early morning snack
5:30–6:30 a.m. Masters swim workout
7:30 a.m. Mini breakfast
10:00 a.m. Mid-morning snack
12:30 p.m. Mini lunch
3:30 p.m. Mid-afternoon snack
4:30–5:30 p.m. Run workout
6:30 p.m. Mini dinner
10 p.m. Bedtime

Note the spacing of the meals: They are typically two to three hours apart. Spreading them out evenly helps keep your energy level more constant throughout the day. Notice also that four of the six meals have been consumed by midday. This means we are "front loading" our calories a bit toward the beginning of the day. This makes perfect sense, as this is when our physical and mental needs are at their highest. This simply builds on the old adage: Eat breakfast like a king, lunch like a prince, and dinner like a pauper.

Consistent with this approach, the last of the six meals is at 6:30 p.m., with no food again until the following day. This makes good sense, too. There is no need to take on a lot of calories before bedtime, when we don't need them. Late-night snacks are likely to be stored as fat. One possible exception to this is if you do an evening workout. It may then be helpful to have a light healthy snack after your evening workout.

With a 10 p.m. bedtime, this may mean up to three hours without food after dinner. This is one of the most challenging time periods of weight management. It's so easy to have a late-night snack that will put you over on calories for the day. If you find it helps to hold you over, a small snack of 100 calories or fewer between dinner and bedtime is fine, but be careful not to allow this to lead to a late-night calorie binge.

If you find evening snacking to be a challenge, consider drinking water after dinner to help suppress your appetite. Another strategy is to brush your teeth right after dinner. When we brush our teeth it sort of tells us that we are done eating for the day.

There are many fans of the six-meals-a-day approach, and there are several versions of it out there. Most agree on the same benefits of this approach. On the Web site FitFAQ.com, editor Jamie Clark lists the following benefits:

- More energy

- Less hunger

- Reduced food cravings

- Controlled blood sugar and insulin production

- Reduced body fat storage

- Maintenance of and increased lean muscle mass

I have personally experienced these benefits, and many of the athletes I work with report them as well.

Do I Need to Count Calories?

Counting calories definitely helps! Each person's body has a certain unique number of calories it needs to maintain its current weight. To sort of state the obvious: If you consume less than this amount over time, you tend to lose weight. If you consume more than this amount over time, you tend to gain weight.

Through years of trial and error, 2,400 calories per day seems to be the amount that maintains my weight, net of training. In other words: If I did no training and just did normal daily activities, my weight would remain fairly constant if I consumed 2,400 calories per day.

Furthermore I have found, through trial and error, that if I eat about 500 fewer calories per day (2,400 − 500 = 1,900 calories), I tend to lose weight at a rate of about one pound per week. Likewise, if I eat about 500 calories more than this amount per day (2,400 + 500 = 2,900 calories), I tend to gain weight at the same rate of about one pound per week.

If you can determine what your unique calorie maintenance number is, you can have a great deal of control over your weight. Put yourself in the position of being able to adjust your weight over time by adjusting your daily calorie intake. The technical term for this is *basal metabolic rate* (BMR). In layman's terms, this is the amount of energy your body uses just to keep it functioning. While I originally determined my unique BMR through trial and error, there are many Web sites that can help you to estimate yours, and this may be a good place to start.

Let's say you had your best racing year ever last season, and you were competing at a body weight of 160 pounds. With this year's racing season only two months away, you find you've gained some weight and are now weighing in at 168 pounds. You decide you want to safely reduce to your "race weight." Well, no problem. If you know your calorie needs per my example above, you can make that simple 500 calorie adjustment per day and will gradually lose about one pound a week. In merely eight weeks you should be right down around your "race weight."

Why is it a good idea to lose weight gradually as opposed to losing it quickly? My personal experience has been that if you lose the weight very gradually, you are far more likely to keep the weight off. What's more, often when individuals lose weight rapidly, they feel weak and some even report a higher risk of illness as a result. Finally, rapid weight loss tends to take the good with the bad. When we lose too quickly we are far more likely to lose good lean muscle along with our unwanted excess fat. So always play it safe. If you want to lose weight, do it gradually and safely and under the supervision of a qualified professional.

Is It Okay to Eat Out at Restaurants?

It is okay to eat out, but unless you are very disciplined and have a thorough knowledge of exactly how many calories are in most types of foods, it's best to eat out in moderation. The reality is that if you eat at a restaurant more than a couple of times a week, it is almost impossible to know how many calories you are consuming. There are usually so many hidden calories in restaurant foods. My suggestion is to limit yourself to restaurants no more than two times per week and to try your best to make good food choices when you do.

If you find yourself eating out more often, consider the following tips:

- Limit or eliminate your consumption of alcohol. Hydrate well before and during your meal with water or seltzer with lemon or lime.

- Start your meal with a salad with light oil and vinegar, as opposed to a high-calorie salad dressing.

- Order simple main dishes without a lot of mystery ingredients (with hidden calories).

- Avoid sauces, especially those made with cream, butter, or other high-calorie ingredients.

- Avoid fried foods in favor of grilled or baked foods.

Is It Necessary to Become Organized with Your Nutrition?

While it is not essential to completing an Iron-distance triathlon, if you are serious about maximizing your performance, I encourage you to embrace a serious approach to your eating habits and nutrition.

Athletes often tell me they are discouraged because their weight is not where they would like it to be. When I ask them what they are doing to become leaner, they often tell me they are "trying to lose weight." I have learned that this is just a catch phrase. What it really means is that they are "hoping to lose weight" through training and "watching what they eat." But they are not focusing on how much they are actually eating—that is, they are not focusing on their specific calorie intake.

When I ask these athletes how many calories they are consuming, they throw out a calorie number. With a little probing I usually find that they really don't have any idea. With a little more probing, I often find they are consuming many hidden calories that they had completely forgotten about. I jokingly refer to this as "snack amnesia."

People fall victim to snack amnesia in many ways. It was someone's birthday in the office, so they had a piece of cake. They spent several hours tailgating before the football game. They went out to a big dinner with a client. They went out for drinks and snacks after work with coworkers. It's easy to forget situations like this, but chances are that unless you really focus on your calorie intake, they will continue to pop up during the week, and you will regularly take in a lot more calories than you think you are. Remember: An average of just 500 calories extra per day can lead to gaining one pound a week.

One of my favorite excuses is, "I have children, so I have to have cookies and ice cream around the house." Of course this is not true. Why would we want to teach our children that ice cream and cookies should be part of our normal diet? Instead, these should be "reward foods," which we will discuss later in this chapter.

Because it's so easy to fall into snack amnesia, I encourage you to dial in on exactly how many calories you consume and how many you burn during training.

What About Calories Burned While Training?

Figuring out the calories you need to sustain normal activity seems easy enough, but this does not take into account the calories used in training. This complicates the calculation a bit, and this is where most athletes go off track.

If you need to consume a specific number of calories per day to maintain your weight, net of training, how much do you need to consume to compensate for your training? This question becomes even more complicated when you consider that you do different types of training on different days, with varying durations and intensity levels. It is not as if each day you burn the same number of calories.

For example: If you need 2,400 calories per day to maintain your weight, and you used 600 calories on a particular day of training, then you would need to consume 3,000 calories per day (2,400 + 600 = 3,000 calories) to maintain your weight and some amount less than that to lose weight. Since I do different activities every day, I have developed a range of calories for each of the three sports and I estimate my calories based on the duration of the activity and my perception of the intensity of the workout.

Following are the calorie ranges that I find work best for me:

- Swim: 500 to 700 calories per hour

- Bike: 700 to 900 calories per hour

- Run: 900 to 1,100 calories per hour

These ranges have worked well for me over the years and have helped me to control my weight. But, just like determining your own unique calorie needs, you need to determine calorie ranges for the training activities you participate in.

For example: If I swam a very high intensity one-hour masters swim session in the morning and then ran a very light one-hour run in the late afternoon, I might assign 700 calories for the swim and 900 calories for the run. This would mean that I would apply a combined negative 1,600 calories (700 + 900 = 1,600 calories) to my calorie totals for the day, to compensate for my training activity. If my estimates are correct, and my needed calorie consumption to maintain weight is a net 2,400, to maintain my same weight I would try to consume about 4,000 calories that day (2,400 + 1,600 = 4,000). It's at times like this that I realize how great it is to be an endurance athlete! Think about it: 4,000 guilt-free calories!

This approach has worked well for me over the years. I have kept track of my consumed calories and my estimated calories used in the three sports, and as a result, I have developed a good feel for what my calorie and training needs are in order to get my weight where I want it to be, to be healthy, and to race my best. While it takes a little work, I suggest this approach to any athlete trying to achieve a healthy lean race weight.

There are many resources available to help you estimate your own calorie ranges for your activities. A good example of one is diet4uonline.com.

Balanced Calories

All calorie sources are not the same. Carbohydrates, proteins, and fats each do different things, and all play a role in a healthy diet. While I often hear about "protein diets," "low-fat diets," and many other trendy approaches, I have found that a well-balanced healthy diet and proper portion control have always worked best for me as an athlete.

What does the United States Department of Agriculture (USDA) consider to be a healthy diet? Their Dietary Guidelines for Americans describe a healthy diet as one that does the following:

- Emphasizes fruits, vegetables, whole grains, and fat-free or low-fat milk and milk products

- Includes lean meats, poultry, fish, beans, eggs, and nuts

- Is low in saturated fats, trans fats, cholesterol, salt (sodium), and added sugars.

Probably none of these points surprises you. But after years of trial and error, I find these guidelines fit right in with the optimal approach to eating for me, which includes healthy carbohydrates, protein, and fats. Only when I am getting all three of these, in the right ratios, do I feel my best and perform at my best as an athlete.

Many nutrition experts say that a diet made up of 40 percent carbohydrates, 30 percent protein, and 30 percent fat works best for most people. While my best ratio seems to be a little different (more like 50 percent carbohydrates, 25 percent protein, and 25 percent fat), I have found that most athletes I work with are fairly close to the suggested ratio. So if you are looking for a good place to start, I would recommend beginning with the 40-30-30 ratio.

While I find that maintaining my ratio on a daily basis keeps my energy level at its highest, I feel even better still when each of my six small meals includes the same ratio as well. Now, it's almost impossible and certainly not worth the effort to calculate this exactly for every little meal, but I find that if I can at least include all three nutrients in each meal, with the goal of hitting my 50-25-25 ratio for the entire day, I remain at the absolute most consistent level of energy throughout the day.

Hydration

This one is big! Hydration is so important, and I see too many athletes not giving it the attention it deserves. We all know how critically important a proper hydration level is to athletic performance, but for some reason hydration only becomes a focus around race time. Hydration needs to be part of your diet every day. It keeps you feeling well and ready to get the most out of every training session. Even a modest 2 percent dehydration that occurs prior to, or during, exercise can negatively impact your performance.

Often when athletes tell me they are feeling a little blah, the first thing I ask them about is their hydration. And often I find they have not been drinking as much fluid as they should be drinking for their activity levels. We then make a correction, and it's amazing how often it does the trick.

Now if I am feeling a little blah, the first thing I do is grab a nice cool bottle of water from the refrigerator. Next to sleep, it's one of the very best things you can do to get the most out of your training. In fact most times when athletes tell me they are feeling a little fatigued and run-down, I suggest they take the day off, get some extra sleep, and get fully hydrated.

One other great benefit of maintaining proper hydration levels is that most people find if they are well-hydrated, they feel less hungry. This can be very helpful if you want to keep cravings under control, as dehydration can often cause a sensation of hunger.

Reward Foods

Needless to say there are certain foods that aren't that good for us and should not be part of our regular diet. We all have certain foods that are hard for us to stay away from, despite the fact we know we should. Here's how I deal with this, as do many of my coached athletes. Instead of cutting these foods out of my diet completely, I designate them as "reward foods." In other words, instead of deciding I will never have these foods again, which is a promise I know I cannot keep, I treat myself to them only as a reward for certain accomplishments.

One of my food weaknesses is french fries—the saltier the better. I don't want french fries to be part of my regular diet, but I doubt I can say good-bye to them forever. So french fries are one of my primary reward foods.

After a good race I usually have french fries as part of my post-race celebration. Sometimes I even hit the drive-through window on the way home. This approach keeps them in their proper place in my overall diet, and I enjoy them even more when I eat them because it feels like an extra celebration.

I often joke with my athletes about my "twenty-four-hour rule." After a good race they are allowed to eat "reward foods" for the next twenty-four hours. While I mean it half-jokingly, an interesting benefit usually occurs with this approach. After eating glazed doughnuts for twenty-four hours straight after a big race, the athlete gets pretty sick of them and is more than happy to get back into training and wait until after the next big race to eat them again.

Resources

As I mentioned before, please consider what I have said here about nutrition and hydration, but before changing your own eating habits, consult a nutrition expert and always be safe and proceed with caution.

Here are just some of the resources available to help you with nutrition planning:

- www.usda.gov

- www.cnpp.usda.gov

- www.foodsafety.gov

- www.weightwatchers.com

AN IRONFIT MOMENT

Whenever I talk to one of my coached athletes about nutrition, they often ask: "Can you just give me an example of what you eat?" While I understand that this is a tempting approach, because it is a lot simpler, it's important to remember that the optimal diet for anyone is unique to that individual. That is why I suggest working with professionals to determine what is best for you. But to give an example of how I approach this, below is a typical day for me based on my targeted net calories of 2,400; my estimated range for calories burned; and my target ratio of 50 percent carbohydrates, 25 percent protein, and 25 percent fat.

5:00 a.m.: Wake Up and Early Morning Snack (600 Calories)

- Coffee with skim milk
- Energy drink
- Two energy bars
- GU energy gel
- Water

5:30–6:30 a.m.: Masters Swim Workout (Negative 550 Calories)

- High-intensity one-hour swim utilizes 700 calories
- Energy drink (150 calories)

8:00 a.m.: Mini Breakfast (700 Calories)

- Two slices of oat bran toast with peanut butter and jelly
- Low-fat yogurt
- Pear or banana
- Water

10:30 a.m.: Mid-Morning Snack (450 Calories)

- Apple slices with almond butter
- Cottage cheese with pineapple
- Water

12:30 p.m.: Mini Lunch (750 Calories)

- Spinach salad with grilled chicken, feta cheese, peppers, carrots, walnuts, and red wine vinegar dressing
- Whole wheat crackers
- Water

3:30 p.m.: Mid- to Late-Afternoon Snack (450 Calories)

- Tuna and slices of low-fat cheese on Wasa crackers
- Pretzels
- Coffee with skim milk
- Water

5:00–6:00 p.m.: Run Workout (Negative 750 Calories)

- Moderate-intensity one-hour run utilizes 900 calories
- Energy drink (150 calories)

6:30 p.m.: Mini Dinner (750 Calories)

- Whole wheat pasta with shrimp, almonds, chickpeas, and parsley
- Steamed broccoli with lemon and oil
- Green salad with tomatoes and onions
- Water

10:00 p.m.: Bedtime

Calculations:

4,000 calories consumed
1,600 calories utilized in training
2,400 net calories

TAKE ACTION CHALLENGE

The following is a sample daily calorie worksheet. Once you have consulted a nutrition expert, use this worksheet each day to determine your net calories for the day:

Athlete: _____

Date: _____

Daily Net Calorie Target: _____

Calories Consumed: _____

    Meal #1: _____

    Meal #2: _____

    Meal #3: _____

    Meal #4: _____

    Meal #5: _____

    Meal #6: _____

    Total Calories Consumed: _____

Calories Utilized: _____

    Training Session #1: _____

    Training Session #2: _____

    Training Session #3: _____

    Total Calories Utilized: _____

Net Calories for Day: _____

CHAPTER 19

Recovery, Maintenance Training, and Beyond

"If you have the courage to begin, you have the courage to succeed."

—*David Viscott*

Recovery and the Morning After

Once you have completed an Iron-distance triathlon, there are specific things you should (and shouldn't) do to speed your recovery, maintain your base fitness level, and ready yourself for your next goal. I will start with the week after the race.

- **Day One:** Complete rest. Assuming you have no injury that requires attention, try to walk as normally as possible. This includes walking up and down stairs, which is usually somewhat uncomfortable the day after a race. Consider getting a massage to help you feel better and to speed your recovery.

  Otherwise, celebrate! You have accomplished something few will ever attempt. It's easy to pick apart your race, but don't. If you want to improve upon what you did, great. The journey will continue. But for today, celebrate and be proud of what you have accomplished. You are a member of a very exclusive club.

  Spend some of the day thanking those who made it possible. Let them all know how much you appreciate their sacrifices and share your victory with them.

  Eat healthy. Your body needs good fuel to repair itself. And while you are probably sick of energy drinks, try to stay hydrated.

One other reminder: When I say celebrate, I don't mean drink alcoholic beverages. Hold off on that urge for a while, or at least drink very moderately. It's not what your body wants right now.

- **Day Two:** This is often your travel day. Take another day off from training, as packing, loading, driving, flying, etc., will really make you feel all of those sore spots from the race. Try to go as easy as possible and be extra careful when lifting and loading luggage. Your muscles are probably going to be sore and stiff.

- **Day Three:** Time to get back on the horse. A moderate level of activity will actually help speed your recovery at this point. I recommend an easy 30-minute spin on your bike or an easy 30-minute swim, or both.

- **Day Four:** Take a longer easy spin on the bike (45 to 60 minutes) and an easy swim if you did not have one the day before.

- **Day Five:** Attempt an easy 20-minute jog if you feel up to it. Even if it feels good, wait at least a day before running any farther, and only increase the duration very gradually.

After these first five days, I recommend that you move into an off-season maintenance program. This should be a period of at least 1 month in which you only do aerobic exercise before going back into training for a specific race. It's good to "cycle down" your training for a while after an Iron-distance race. It gives you an opportunity to fully recover, both physically and mentally, and to recharge your batteries for your next challenge.

I do not recommend complete rest. You will lose a great deal of your hard-earned conditioning and injury resistance, and your comeback will be difficult. At a minimum I recommend 5 hours per week of training and at least two sessions each of swimming, cycling, and running.

The following is a sample minimum maintenance program:

Monday: Rest day
Tuesday: 45-minute aerobic run

Wednesday:	30-minute swim (focus on technique), plus 30 minutes of strength training
Thursday:	45-minute aerobic bike
Friday:	30-minute swim (focus on technique), plus 30 minutes of strength training
Saturday:	90-minute aerobic bike
Sunday:	60-minute aerobic run

Total weekly hours: 6

This type of program will help you to fully recover and maintain a good level of fitness. You will then be well-positioned to reenter the Base Phase of training, when you so decide.

PIB

It's Tuesday morning and you're back at the office. Only yesterday you were at the awards dinner celebrating one of the greatest accomplishments of your life with your family, friends, and thousands of exhilarated fellow triathletes. Only 2 days ago you accomplished something so remarkable that you once thought it impossible. For the past 12 months you have trained for several hours every day and lived a balancing act that few can understand. For more years than you can remember, you have dreamed about completing an Iron-distance triathlon and wondered if it was something that you could ever find the strength to accomplish.

Through all this, there were days of injury and setback, days when it appeared to be all over and the dream was dead. But you kept fighting back, kept overcoming the many obstacles along the way that life most certainly brings. In the end, you somehow prevailed. Your strength and perseverance proved stronger than all of the obstacles. You accomplished something truly great, something that most will only ever dream about.

But now it's the day after. While you may have been at the mountaintop yesterday, today you find yourself back in the valley. Sure, your coworkers all have their congratulations for you, maybe even a little gathering in the conference room with coffee and bagels to welcome you back. But once you return to your desk, you find it overflowing with work. You have a record number of emails. Your boss, who was very understanding of your shorter work hours during your key training phase, is now ready for a little payback.

As each day goes by, your trip to the mountaintop seems further and further in your past. The normality of ordinary life has taken over. Your great accomplishment seems like a distant memory, and the great goal and purpose you had been living with for so long is now gone.

Don't be concerned. These feelings are common among Iron-distance competitors, especially among first timers. In fact, the response is so common that veterans jokingly refer to it as "PIB": the Post-Iron-distance Blues.

Following are my tips, together with the suggestions of several Ironmen, on how to beat the Post-Iron-distance Blues.

1. **Keep the Celebration Going:** Most agree: Don't let the celebration end at the awards ceremony. Remember to mark your success with your own special celebration, or a series of celebrations, worthy of your accomplishment:

> *"Most importantly, take the time to celebrate your success with your friends and family. Go out to dinner, eat ice cream, do all of the fun things you may have been neglecting. Put your finish line photo on your desk."*
>
> —MELANIE FINK

> *"Eat chocolate, drink beer or whatever 'evils' you had limited yourself on your hard road to Ironman."*
>
> —ANDREW JONES

2. **Plan Events in Advance:** One great way to avoid the potential void after your race is to plan ahead and eliminate the void in advance.

> *"Before Ironman, I start planning the weeks afterwards. I plan to do something I've wanted to do but haven't had time. I set it up before I leave for Ironman. Then after Ironman, I have something to look forward to."*
>
> —KATY ROBERTS

"Schedule a party at your house and start planning the menu and the guest list before you leave for Ironman, so when you get home you can just jump into it."

—JODI LEE ALPER

3. **Put a Race on the Calendar:** Once a major goal has been accomplished, one of the best things to replace it with is another goal of equal worth.

Andrew Jones recommends a two-part racing strategy. While Andrew has already committed to another Iron-distance race next year, he also recommends doing "a short race for fun, 2 to 4 weeks after the Ironman." Andrew adds, "It's amazing how fit you are and how easy an Olympic-distance race is after an Ironman."

"I set another racing goal for the future—preferably in a couple months, so not to put too much pressure on myself, but to know it's there."

—KATY ROBERTS

4. **Dedicate Yourself to Balance:** While a new goal is greatly beneficial, sometimes we can best deal with the initial post-Iron-distance period by mending some fences. Having been so focused on training for a long period, we may not have given our family, friends, or employers their fair share of our time. We may even feel guilty for this, which contributes to our blue feelings.

"Take time to thank all of the people in your life who helped make that day a success. Also, volunteer at a local race or find a way to help someone else achieve their goal."

—MELANIE FINK

*"Do all of the things at work and in your personal life
that you put off during your training weeks."*

—JODI LEE ALPER

*"Take a weekend break with your family and
friends and indulge."*

—ANDREW JONES

5. **Be Easy on Yourself:** Give your body and mind a well-deserved rest. Allow yourself to rejuvenate. And if after trying all of the above, you still feel those blue feelings creeping in, don't be too hard on yourself. Realize that your feelings are normal, and most triathletes experience them at some level.

*"I think what helped me this year is to keep reminding
myself that my body went through a lot with training
and racing, and now it's time to be good to my body. I give
it a gift, sleep in, massages. . . . When I do get blue afterwards,
I tell myself that it's okay. We Ironmen all go through PIB.
I'll get through this too."*

—KATY ROBERTS

*"Keep life in perspective . . . I reflect, I use it as a new
learning experience."*

—ADRIAN JONES

Maintenance Training

The meaning of "maintenance training" varies greatly from athlete to athlete. Many consider maintenance training to be casual training of low volume and low intensity. They do this for several months while they "rest up" for the coming season. While this may work for some, for many this maintenance period is actually a slow process of deconditioning. They start the next season at a relatively low fitness level, and with the same strengths and weaknesses they had the previous year.

- **Target Weaknesses**

Consider this alternative. Decrease your training volume to a comfortable off-season level, but then select two "weaknesses" to focus on. Make it your off-season goal to improve in these two areas substantially before the start of next season. Build these goals into your off-season training program.

Sure, you will still have to build up volume at the start of next season to be ready to race, but if you are successful with this approach, you will have two new weapons in your arsenal when you do. I have worked with many

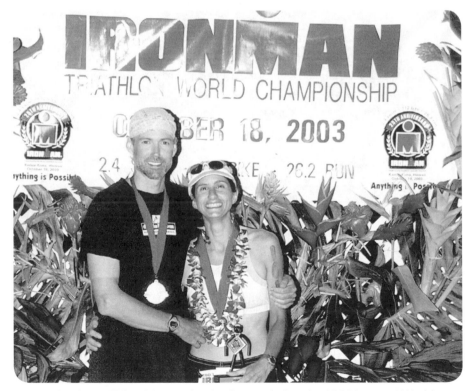

Don and Melanie Fink celebrate after both completing the 2003 Ironman World Championships.
Photo Credit: Verismile.

Iron-distance triathletes who have scaled back their training by 50% to 5 to 10 hours per week (from a peak of 10 to 20) and have been able to make substantial progress on two of their weaknesses in the off-season. Let's look at a couple of examples.

- **"The Runner"**: Many triathletes come from a running background and their swim tends to be their weakness. And many of them put swimming on the backburner during the off-season in favor of running road races (their strength!). What they tend to find at the start of next season is that swimming is still their weakness (and weaker than usual), and running is still their strength. Nothing much has changed.

  How about this instead? What if The Runner joins a Masters swim team and trains for and competes in Masters events over the winter? Sure, she may feel a little out of her element, but by next spring she will surely be a better and more confident swimmer. Plus she will probably find the change of pace refreshing.

- **"The Swimmer"**: Yes, this works in reverse. I often advise the strong swimmers I coach to develop their running skills over the winter. A great way to do this is to focus a good portion of the athlete's reduced workout time on training for and racing in winter road races. For long-course athletes, we usually make it our off-season goal to set new personal records in the half marathon and marathon; my Olympic-distance athletes target the 5K and 10K. This is a great approach: Swimmers utilizing this strategy usually enter their next triathlon season as faster and more confident runners.

Training Tips for the Off-Season

Here are some more tips for making the most of the off-season.

- **Swim Technique Review**

The beginning of the off-season is a perfect time to work on your swimming technique. Have your swimming videotaped and analyzed by an expert. If there are major corrections to be made, this is the best time to do it. After your technique flaws have been identified, you may want to ask an expert to recommend corrective drills. If so, work exclusively on these drills for 4 to 8 weeks. Don't do any "regular" swimming during this time; you want to break those bad habits, not repeat them. After this drills-only period, go back for re-taping and analysis and determine your progress. I have worked with athletes who have followed this strategy and were successful in raising their swim to a new level over the off-season.

For many athletes, an expert review of cycling or running technique (or both) can be equally beneficial.

• Address Injuries

If you have had chronic aches and pains that you have been procrastinating over, now is the time to deal with them. Go see the appropriate specialist(s) and get some good advice on how best to recover. If you need rest, now is the time.

• Strength and Core Training

If your strength and core training program has gotten stale or has just fallen off your priority list, now is the time to get it going again. Start with the Strength and Core Training Programs for the maintenance phase (in Chapter 8 and 9) or have a knowledgeable multisport coach design a new program for you that freshens up your routine and gets your enthusiasm going again.

• Indoor Cycling

Now is a great time to work on your cycling power. While indoor training has some drawbacks (e.g., boredom), there are also some big advantages to working with your bike indoors on the trainer. You can control your resistance, cadence, and heart rate much more easily and really put some quality work in. For most of the athletes I coach, I recommend shorter, more intense cycling sessions in the off-season to build power. It is generally not necessary to do a lot of volume, as there will be time for that later. Try some of the great cycling videos available to liven up and bring focus to your indoor power-building sessions (see Appendix B—Resources).

What Comes Next in Your Journey?

You have achieved your Iron Dream.

It was a doable challenge. It was a worthy challenge. It has helped you to grow as a person, and expanded your sense of what is possible in your life. It will change the way the people in your life feel about you, and how you feel about yourself.

Now, what do you do next? Virtually all Iron-distance triathletes agree that it is a life-changing experience. A few may return to "normal" life and carry on pretty much as they did before. For most, however, the Iron-distance serves as the starting point of living and viewing life in a new way. They may go back to the life they lived before, but things will be different—and they will be better.

One of the lessons you learn when you cross your first Iron-distance finish line is that it's not really a finish line. It's just a milestone on a much greater journey. Now you know that what may at first seem impossible is not. Now you see obstacles and "failures" for what they are: opportunities to learn and grow. Now you will choose action over inaction. You will always commit to your dreams.

Appendix A
Suggested Reading

The books listed here have proven very helpful to me over the years, and have provided a great deal of information to me as I compiled my research. They may prove useful to you as well.

- *The Achievement Zone: 8 Skills for Winning All the Time from Playing Field to Boardroom.* Shane Murphy, Ph.D. G. S. Putnam's Sons. 1996.
- *Bicycling Magazine's Complete Guide to Riding and Racing Techniques.* Fred Matheny. Rodale Press. 1989.
- *Core Performance.* Mark Verstegen and Pete Williams. Rodale. 2004.
- *The Core Program.* Peggy W. Brill, P.T. with Gerald Secor Couzens. Bantam Books. 2001.
- *Dave Scott's Triathlon Training.* Dave Scott. Simon & Schuster, Inc. 1986.
- *Diamonds Under Pressure: Five Steps to Turning Adversity into Success.* Barry F. Farber. Berkley Books. 1998.
- *Eating for Endurance.* Dr. Philip Maffetone. David Barmore Productions. 1999.
- *Embracing Your Potential: Steps to Self-Discovery, Balance, and Success in Sports, Work, and Life.* Terry Orlick, PhD. Human Kinetics. 1998.
- *The Essential Swimmer.* Steve Tarpinian. Lyons & Burford. 1996.
- *The Essential Triathlete.* Steven Jonas. The Lyons Press. 1996.
- *Going Long.* Joe Friel and Gordon Byrn. Velo Press. 2003.
- *How to Eat, Move and Be Healthy.* Paul Chek. C.H.E.K. Institute Publishing. 2004.
- *The Inner Athlete: Realizing Your Fullest Potential.* Dan Millman. Stillpoint Publishing. 1994.
- *Instant Relief: Tell Me Where It Hurts and I'll Tell You What to Do.* Peggy W. Brill, P.T. with Susan Suffes. Bantam Books. 2003.

- *Lifelong Success Triathlon: Training for Masters.* Henry Ash & Barbara Warren. Meyer & Meyer Sport (UK) Ltd. 2003.
- *Lifestyle & Weight Management Consultant Manual.* American Council on Exercise. Richard T. Cotton. 1996.
- *Mark Allen's Total Triathlete.* Mark Allen with Bob Babbitt. Contemporary Books. 1984.
- *In Pursuit of Excellence: How to Win in Sport and Life Through Mental Training.* Terry Orlick, PhD. Leisure Press. 1990.
- *Personal Training Manual—The Resource for Fitness Professionals.* Richard T. Cotton. American Council on Exercise. 1996.
- *Program Design for Personal Trainers: Bridging Theory into Application.* Douglas S. Brooks, MS. Human Kinetics. 1997.
- *Serious Training for Endurance Athletes.* Rob Sleamaker & Ray Browning. Human Kinetics. 1996.
- *Starting Out Triathlon: Training for Your First Competition.* Paul Huddle and Roch Frey, with Bob Babbitt. Meyer & Meyer Sport (UK) Ltd. 2003.
- *Time Saving Training for Multisport Athletes.* Rick Niles. Human Kinetics. 1997.
- *Total Immersion.* Terry Laughlin and John Delves. Simon & Schuster, Inc. 1996.
- *The Total Triathlon Almanac-4.* Tony Svensson. The Trimarket Company. 1998.
- *Training and Racing Biathlons.* Mark Sisson. Primal Urge Press. 1989.
- *Training Lactate Pulse-Rate.* Peter G. J. M. Janssen. Polar Electro Oy. 1987.
- *Training Plans for Multisport Athletes.* Gale Bernhardt. Velo Press. 2000.
- *The Triathlete's Training Bible.* Joe Friel. Velo Press. 1998.
- *Triathlon 101: Essentials for Multisport Success.* John Mora. Human Kinetics. 1999.
- *Triathlon Training Book.* Mark Sisson. Macmillan. 1983.
- *Triathloning for Ordinary Mortals.* Steven Jonas, M. D. W. W. Norton. 1986.

Appendix B
Resources

Special Book Contributors

Ryan Grote
The Running Company
108 Nassau Street
Princeton, NJ 08542
(609) 252–9110
www.therunningcompany.net

Paul Levine
Signature Cycles
2 Grandview Rd
Central Valley, NY 10917
T (845) 928-3060
F (845) 928-3061
email: Info@signaturecycles.com
www.signaturecycles.com

Dr. John M. Schneider
159 East 74th Street
New York, NY 10021
(212) 249-7790
schnidu@hotmail.com
www.activerelease.com

Meg Waldron
Certified Neuromuscular Therapist and Fitness Trainer
Megafit1@aol.com

Jan Wanklyn
Massage/Performance Care
Jan_w@aol.com

Coaching Resources

- Don Fink (www.donfink.com)
- Mark Allen (www.markallenonline.com)
- Gordo Byrn (www.coachgordo.com)
- Troy Jacobson (www.coachtroy.com)
- Paul Huddle & Roche Fry (www.multisports.com)
- Dave Scott (www.davescottinc.com)

Clinics and Workshops

- Multisports. Paul Huddle & Roche Fry. (www.multisports.com)
- Movement U. Jessi Stensland. (gojessi.com)
- Total Immersion. Terry Laughlin. (www.totalimmersion.net)
- Total Training University. Steve Tarpinian. (www.swimpower.com)

Video Resources

- Ironman Race Videos (1991 to Present). Ironman Store. (www.ironman.com)
- Spinervals & Runnervals. Troy Jacobson. (www.coachtroy.com)
- Swim Power and Swim Power II Synergistic Swimming. Steve Tarpinian. (www.swimpower.com)
- Total Immersion. (www.totalimmersion.net)

Appendix C
Selected Iron-Distance Race Links

Following are Web site links for various Iron-Distance Races:

- www.Ironman.com
- www.TriFind.com
- www.USATriathlon.org
- www.raceforum.com

Appendix D
Additional Maximum Heart Rate Estimation Formula

In an article by Paul Keegan ("We Won't Let Him Hurt You") in the February, 1998 issue of *Outside* magazine, the great Mark Allen's (six-time winning of the Ironman World Championships) approach to estimating maximum heart rates is presented:

"Subtract your age from 180, and then adjust that number to reflect your particular circumstances. If you're recovering from a major illness or taking medication, subtract 10; if regular exercise is a hazy memory, subtract 5; if you've been working out consistently for two years or less, stick with 180 minus your age; if you've been exercising without injury for more than two years, add five."

According to Paul Keegan, Mark Allen recommends an aerobic training range of 60% to 80% of the number yielded by this formula.

Index

About the Author

Don Fink is an internationally known triathlon and running coach, and author. Through their business IronFit® (www.IronFit.com), Don and his wife Melanie have trained hundreds of athletes on four continents to personal best times and breakthrough performances, utilizing their innovative training approaches.

In addition to being a coach, Don Fink is also an elite athlete. He has raced over 30 Iron-distance triathlons (2.4-mile swim, 112-mile bike, and 26.2-mile run) and has recorded many age group victories and course records. Don's time of 9:08 at the 2004 Ironman Florida is still one of the fastest times recorded by an athlete in the 45–49 age group. Don also placed in the top three overall in the 2002 Ultra Man World Championships (6.2-mile swim, 262-mile bike, and 52.4-mile run) on the Big Island of Hawaii.

He lives in Morris County, New Jersey.